SMART FATS

SMART FATS

How Dietary Fats and Oils Affect Mental, Physical and Emotional Intelligence

MICHAEL A. SCHMIDT

Frog, Ltd
Berkeley, California

Smart Fats:How Dietary Fats and Oils Affect Mental, Physical and Emotional Intelligence

Published by Frog, Ltd.

Frog, Ltd. books are distributed by
North Atlantic Books
P.O. Box 12327
Berkeley, CA 94712

Cover and book design by Andrea DuFlon
Illustrations by Michael Bryant
Printed in the United States of America

Library of Congress Cataloging-in-Publication Data

Schmidt, Michael A., 1958–
    Smart Fats: How Dietary Fats and Oils Affect Mental, Physical and
    Emotional Intelligence
    Michael A. Schmidt.
      p.   cm.
    Includes bibliographical references and index.
    ISBN 1-883319-62-5
    1. Neurochemistry. 2. Fatty acids in human nutrition. 3. Brain-Physiology.
4. Nervous system—Physiology. I. Title.
QP356.3.S32   1997
612.3'97—dc21   96-37578
                                                         CIP

2 3 4 5 6 7 8 9 / 00 99 98

To Julie, a wellspring of kindness, wisdom, and gentle compassion.

ACKNOWLEDGEMENTS

I would first and foremost like to thank the real pioneers in the field of fatty acids. Without their work, we would not stand in the fascinating place in which we currently find ourselves. Included are Drs. George and Mildred Burr, who are credited with the discovery of essential fatty acids, and Sir John Vane, Prof. Bengt Samulsson, and Prof. Sune Bergstrom for their Nobel Prize-winning work on essential fatty acids. I would like to thank Prof. Hugh Sinclair, Prof. Ulf von Euler, Michael Crawford, Ph.D., Artemis Simopoulos, M.D., Donald Rudin, M.D., David Horrobin, M.D., Jean-Marie Bourré, M.D., Maria Enig, Ph.D., Norman Salem, Ph.D., Ralph Holman, Ph.D., Joseph Hibbeln, M.D., and the many others too numerous to mention.

I would like to thank my colleagues at the Functional Medicine Research Center, especially Buck Levin, Ph.D., Trula Thompson, M.D., Dan Luckazar, M.D., and Connie Brown, M.D. I have deeply appreciated their thoughts, insights, and support. To Jeffrey Bland, Ph.D. I would like to extend a special thanks. His vision, enthusiasm, and ability to tease out the story from a sea of information has been influential in my own professional pursuit. I would also like to thank Leo Galland, M.D., David Perlmutter, M.D., and Patricia Kane, Ph.D. for sharing their very interesting cases and for their thoughtful insights. I am grateful to Gloria Roohr-Heizer, N.D., Virginia Shapiro, D.C., and Lee Ross for their case reports. Also, my thanks to Jay Burgess, Ph.D. and Laura Stevens for sharing their work on ADHD.

I'm grateful to Larry Dossey, M.D. for his thoughts and pioneering ideas, and for his openness and support. My thanks also to Andrew Weil, M.D. A special thanks goes to my friend, colleague, and mentor Sidney Baker, M.D. Sydney's ability to teach by metaphor, allegory, and anecdote make even the most crusty subjects come alive with richness and flavor. His gentleness, insightfullness, and respect for all things makes him one of the true wisdom keepers of our time.

To two of my mentors: Alexander Melientev, M.D., Chairman of the Department of Internal Medicine at Russian State Medical University. He is among the most inspirational instructors and kind human beings I have known. To Yvgeny Gusev, M.D., Chairman of the Department of Neurology and Neurosurgery at Russian State Medical University. I appreciate his gentle and insightful way of teaching.

I am grateful to Dr. Michael Bryant for his creative work on the illustrations. To Lindy Hough and Richard Grossinger at North Atlantic Books for their support and understanding as I attempted to convey the depth and scope of this very provocative story. To Virginia Baker, for her help in giving this book clarity and consistency. To Anastasia McGhee of North Atlantic Books, whose nurturing support and sensitivity softens the process of bringing a book to fruition.

As with each of my endeavors, my greatest thanks goes out to my wife Julie, who is a consistent source of balance, insight, and honesty. Her strength, wisdom, and loving support is an inspiration to me and a gift to all who cross her path.

To my boys I extend a special thanks and debt of gratitude. They have been my true teachers in the way of the heart. While telling a fascinating story to the world may yield personal rewards, it is their love that truly matters most.

AUTHOR'S NOTE

This book contains a discussion of nutrients that are known to be important in brain structure and function. Though it contains many reviews from the scientific literature, comments about specific nutrients in therapy have not been evaluated by the Food and Drug Administration.

Anyone using this book should do so with full knowledge that there is not yet a consensus of opinion regarding interpretation of the scientific data in this field. The evidence is compelling with regard to the role of certain nutrient compounds in improving brain function. However, opinions may exist that are different than those of the author. For this reason, it is important that you consider all relevant viewpoints and review the relevant data for yourself. Moreover, before attempting to utilize information contained in this book, it is advisable to consult your licensed health care professional. You and your physician or licensed health care professional must take full responsibility for the uses made of this book.

A NOTE ABOUT DHA AND DHEA

Throughout this book, I describe a number of fatty acids that influence brain function. One of the most important among these is DHA, or docosahexaenoic acid. It is important that the reader not confuse the fatty acid DHA with the steroid hormone DHEA. DHEA stands for dehydroepiandrosterone. It is not a fat or dietary substance, but the most abundant steroid hormone in the body. It is the precursor of estrogen, testosterone, and other hormones.

DHA on the other hand, is a dietary fatty acid found in cold water fish and some algae. The brain has an absolute structural requirement for this fatty acid. DHA is thus used therapeutically to provide the brain with the necessary fatty acids to function properly.

DHEA is a hormone/drug that should be used with guidance under professional supervision. DHA is a fatty acid that should be a part of everyone's diet

CONTENTS

PART IV: GETTING THE BRAIN FATS YOU NEED: FOOD AND SUPPLEMENT GUIDE

FOREWORD

Over the past twenty years, most informed consumers have become aware of the simple nutritional story that "excessive dietary fats are bad for one's health." In both laboratory and clinical research, scientists have proved that individuals who consume too much fat are at risk for many degenerative diseases—among them heart disease, adult onset diabetes and some forms of cancer. This research has been implemented by government public health agencies and the food industry to urge and help consumers limit dietary fat intake, in an effort to reduce risk to these diseases.

A more recent body of data suggests that we must be cautious, however, in excessively reducing all fats in the diet, because some fats are essential to our health. These essential fatty acids cannot be manufactured by the body and are critically important in maintaining brain function, a strong immune system, and the proper workings of the heart.

Dr. Michael Schmidt makes the most compelling argument to date on how the essential fats affect the performance of the brain's operations. The author of three previous books on the immune system and nutrition, Dr. Schmidt brings twenty years of teaching and clinical experience to this new aspect of how health is determined by nutrition.

In *Beyond Antibiotics,* Dr. Schmidt described a comprehensive approach to improving the immune system. In *Healing Childhood Ear Infections,* he applied this approach to the leading condition from which young children suffer. In *Tired of Being Tired,* Dr. Schmidt showed how to apply a nutritional approach to the management of chronic fatigue and low energy, and how to tell other similar conditions from CFS. These books have helped many thousands of children and adults to recovery and improved health.

Smart Fats is another book of the same order of magnitude. It describes, in very readable fashion, how reducing "bad fats" and increasing "good fats" can determine the quality of memory, concentration, mental acuity, and coordination. We now know that fats and oils determine a vast number of conditions of the brain and the nervous system, ranging from multiple sclerosis to depression to attention deficit disorder. This dietary regulation continues from childhood to old age.

Dr. Schmidt makes clear that how we eat can profoundly influence how our brain operates. This can translate into altered mood, memory, and behavior. Anyone reading this extraordinary book will take away the profound message that we have much more control over our health through proper diet than most of us recognize. Which kind of dietary fats one eats profoundly impacts one's health as the body grows and ages.

Dr. Schmidt's book will make a key contribution to awakening us to these exciting new discoveries in science and medicine, and make these concepts more available to individuals who can then apply them in their lives in effective ways.

Jeffrey S. Bland, Ph.D
HealthComm International
Gig Harbor, Washington

INTRODUCTION

The brain is arguably the most wondrous and complex organ in the human body. It masterfully orchestrates trillions of daily activities—all beneath our conscious awareness. At the same time, it allows us to move our bodies with grace, speed, and power. It allows us to laugh, to cry, and to love. The brain allows us to organize, catalog, and recall vast amounts of information, and to contemplate their meaning.

Most people are astounded to learn what doctors have largely ignored for decades: that the fibers woven to form the tapestry of the brain are composed primarily of fat. In fact, sixty percent of the brain's structure is fatty material. Doctors probably ignored this fact because they thought dietary fat had little influence on the brain. It was believed that the brain was protected against the dietary habits of its owner.

Today we know differently. We've learned that the fat we put in our mouths has a profound influence on the the brain's function. Indeed, the wrong fats and oils can present tremendous problems for the brain. But the right balance of the "right" fats and oils may be one of the most powerful ways to keep the brain functioning at peak efficiency. This knowledge comes at an interesting time because we have become a culture that has learned to hate fat, while, at the same time, consuming fats not conducive to building peak brain function.

We are on the threshold of something exciting. Though I am impressed by the message hidden in the hundreds of scientific papers written on this subject, I am most touched by the moving stories of people whose lives have been forever transformed by precisely targeting their diets with the proper fats and oils:

- A man who overcame paralysis
- A woman who overcame severe depression
- A man who overcame disabling fears
- A boy who was able to walk for the first time after being paralyzed
- A girl, failing school who rose to near the top of her class
- Aggressive children and adults who were transformed to become calm and respectful

Doctors are notoriously cautious about accepting "anecdotal evidence," or stories such as these. But when we add these and other moving stories to the scientific evidence, we are left with a picture that is both exciting and disturbing. Perhaps more than any other nutrient, dietary fat has the power to effect the very nature of who we are.

Since dietary fat effects brain structure and function, we might say that fats and oils effect:

- Learning, memory, and mental intelligence
- Mood, behavior, and emotional intelligence
- Movement, sensation, and physical intelligence

This book will show how the brain's complex "fatty" tapestry is woven and will show the dietary fatty acids that are needed to bring this about.

THE IMPORTANCE OF ENRICHMENT

Throughout this book, we explore the importance of dietary fats and oils in building and maintaining a brain that functions at its peak. There is one issue not discussed within the text of this story that deserves mention, however. This is the issue of enrichment. It has become clear that the brain is able to grow and expand its connections when provided with ongoing stimulation and enrichment. This means that as we use our brain, the richness and extent of its connections improve. In short, an evolving, complex brain depends upon challenging ourselves with diverse experiences.

Any new growth or expansion of nerve cells, however, requires the raw materials of which nerves are made. This includes fatty acids. Whenever we wish to improve brain function we must provide both the raw materials and the stimulation. This means providing the proper balance of fatty acids needed foster brain repair and the proper activity. For example, improving mental function requires that we provide proper nutrition *and* activities that stimulate mental functions such as memory. If we wish to restore function in someone who has problems with coordination or fine motor control, we must provide proper nutrition *and* stimulation of the body region in which we want to improve function.

It has recently been shown (in animals) that the region of the brain associated with memory, the hippocampus, can actually grow new nerve cells. This was once thought impossible. If we add our knowledge of nutrition to such studies we come to the realization that the brain can be improved by providing nutrient materials and a rich and stimulating life.

PEAK PERFORMANCE

This raises exciting possibilities for individuals in good health who wish to boost their level of performance in whatever they do in life. With our knowledge of brain-fats and enrichment, it may be possible to take our personal performance and achievement to new heights. For people with disorders of the brain, it offers tremendous hope that, by effecting the brain's basic fatty structure, its function may be enhanced. It may also be possible to prevent many of the mental difficulties so common as we age.

This book tells a detailed story about the fascinating relationship between what we eat and the function of our most complex organ—the brain. Though I tell a story woven with the thread of nutrition and neurobiology, I realize that we are much more than the sum of our molecules. As you read this book, recognize the power of fats and oils to influence the brain, and to craft a foundation upon which a rich life can be built. Then place it in context with the vast web of life and the mystery that lies hidden within all things.

Michael A. Schmidt
1997

PART I

BREAKING THE CODE AND UNLOCKING THE MYSTERY

CHAPTER 1

USHERING IN A NEW ERA: IMPLICATIONS OF A BRAIN MADE OF FAT

Every novel idea in science passes through three stages.
First people say it isn't true.
Then they say it is true but not important.
And finally they say it's true and important, but not new.
Anonymous

Andrea had been waging a fierce personal battle, which two years of psychotherapy failed to calm. She was plagued by unpredictable outbursts of anger and rage that often left her family and friends in a state of tension. For Andrea, the rise and fall of emotions and the consequences of her actions, at times, made life seem bleak and uncertain. As her chaotic struggles continued, she suffered from spaciness and fine-motor clumsiness. Difficulty with concentration made normal activity increasingly more challenging.

Andrea and her family took their quest for answers to Sidney Baker, M.D., a former professor at Yale School of Medicine. Dr. Baker, a master at finding the hidden story beneath an illness, observed a set of signs that many doctors might overlook. Andrea had a history of "chicken skin" on the backs of her arms. Her feet were constantly painful, dry, and cracked. The skin was shiny in certain places and, in others, was thick and callused with deep painful fissures that sometimes bled.

Dr. Baker reasoned that these "skin signs" were the marks of essential fatty acid insufficiency. He was well aware that fatty acid imbalance can also influence behavior. He ordered a blood profile to test his suspicions and found that Andrea was deficient in omega-3 fatty acids. After two-weeks on fatty acid therapy, her feet became completely normal. Within one month, her unpredictable outbursts of rage and associated behavioral struggles were over.[1] The transformation of Andrea's brain and nervous system through essential fatty acid therapy is not unique, as the following story illustrates.

A young girl had suffered an abdominal wound that caused her to lose portions of her small and large intestines. Because of her damaged digestive tract, she required many months of intravenous feeding to nurture her frail, wounded body back to health. Within one year of the injury, she began to experience a bewildering array of neurological symptoms that seemed unrelated to her injuries. She was plagued by numbness of the hands and feet, loss of sensation, leg pain, blurred vision, tremors of the arm, and decreased vibration sense—all of which are signs of nerve degeneration. Frequent episodes of weakness left her unable to walk for ten to fifteen minutes at a time.

Blood tests revealed that she had somehow become deficient in the omega-3 essential fat, alpha-linolenic acid. When doctors looked at the intravenous solution she had been receiving they noticed a startling discrepancy. The two essential fatty acids, which should normally be present in a one-to-one ratio (1:1), had been given for an entire year in a ratio of one hundred fifteen-to-one (115:1).* The balance became terribly skewed.

Doctors immediately changed feeding preparations, providing a balance of essential fatty acids that was now a more reasonable 6:1. When fatty acid balance was restored to her feeding mixture, "her neurological symptoms disappeared."[2]

This case showed that insufficient amounts of certain dietary fats could create neurological problems and that restoring fatty

---

*The omega-6 to omega-3 ratio was 115:1. A more reasonable ratio would have been 6:1, though there is some argument for using a 1:1 ratio. See Chapter Four for description.

acid balance could rectify them. While a 115:1 ratio of essential fatty acids was far more than one might receive through normal consumption, no matter how horrible the diet, it underscored the fact that tinkering with the fatty acid balance could have a dramatic affect on the brain and nervous system.

These cases raise vital questions about how our brains might be affected by our current dietary habits, ones that are so often nearly devoid of fats critical to the brain. In recent years, we have learned that a normal brain cannot be made without omega-3 fatty acids and, further, that the effect of dietary fats and oils on the brain may be more profound than that of almost any food.

FROM MOOD TO BEHAVIOR: WHEN BRAIN-FATS ARE LOW

The scientific papers surrounding the role of fat and the brain now number in the thousands. For example, doctors in Great Britain found that breast-fed children had IQs that were several points higher than that of bottle-fed children. Breast milk is known to contain the fatty acids critical to brain development, but formula contained none of these fats (prior to 1997).[3]

When scientists studied the brains of people with multiple sclerosis, they found that the brain tissue was very low in important fatty acids such as DHA. They also found low levels of omega-3 fatty acids in blood and almost no omega-3 fatty acids stored in fat tissues.[4]

Doctors in Australia who studied the blood of people with moderate to severe depression found that the balance of essential fatty acids was significantly altered; the level of the omega-3 fatty acids was too low. This adds to a growing body of data suggesting that depression may be closely linked to dietary fat.[5]

Purdue University researchers found that individuals with symptoms of hyperactivity and attention deficit had lower levels of the omega-3 fatty acid DHA in their blood.[6] Behavior and school performance as well as violence and aggression may also show similar links to dietary fatty acids.[7]

Cases have been reported in which learning problems, memory problems, mood disorders, behavior problems, tremors, numbness, developmental delays, seizures, stroke, autism, and other brain-related disorders have been corrected or improved by feeding appropriate fats and oils.

These are only a sample of the the profound effects that fats and oils may have on the brain and nervous system. While there are now scores of scientific papers on the effects of dietary fat on the human brain, years of observation of the animal kingdom have shown that brain structure and function can be affected dramatically when the right balance of fats and oils is not available during critical periods of life. For example:

> **Fatty Acids and Brain Size.** Pups from a large litter had brains that were significantly smaller than those of pups in a small litter. This was presumably because the nutrients, especially fatty acids, were inadequate to meet the demands of the large number of animals. Once the small brain size had been established, no changes could be made in the brain size regardless of fatty acid feeding.[8]

> **Fatty Acids and Brain Cell Numbers.** Animals who consumed low amounts of specific essential fatty acids over three generations experienced an actual drop in the number of brain cells by the third generation.[9] It seems that in the absence of adequate essential fatty acids, the brain does not have enough raw material to make the needed nerve cells.

> **Fatty Acids and Vision.** Primates who consumed low amounts of omega-3 fatty acids prior to conception and during pregnancy had offspring with poor visual acuity. Response to visual stimulation was reduced to only fifty percent of normal in the fatty acid deficient monkeys. The level of the important fatty acid DHA in the brain was only one-sixth of normal in animals that consumed inadequate fatty acids.[10]

> **Fatty Acids and Learning.** Animals consuming inadequate amounts of omega-3 fatty acids had significantly lower amounts of the important fat DHA in their brains than animals consuming a diet rich in these fats. When scientists studied their ability to learn to avoid a threatening situation, the high omega-3 group was 100 percent successful after

only three attempts. In the group fed a low omega-3 diet success was only thirty to forty percent even after the twentieth attempt. The authors concluded, "This indicated that a deficiency in the brain DHA level resulted in a reduction in learning ability."[11]

Taken together, there is a consistent pattern. Specific essential fatty acids are necessary for proper brain development and function.

PROFOUND INFLUENCE

This represents only an introduction into the fascinating story of how fat might affect the function of your brain and nervous system. But the evidence I've shared thus far compels us to question: How is that so simple a family of nutrients, the much maligned fats, has such far-reaching effects on a complex structure like the brain?

Indeed, Dr. Norman Salem, of the National Institutes of Health, has remarked, "This may be the only case in modern day biology where an alteration of the behavior of the whole organism can be reasonably ascribed to a change in structure at the atomic level."[12] In these remarks, Salem implies that simple modification in the structure of a fatty acid has such a profound influence on function of the brain as to affect the spectrum of behavior and functions in which the brain engages—in essence, it has the power to change who we are.

Dr. J. Farquharson seemed to ascribe similar importance when he compared dietary fatty acids such as DHA to genetic influences with respect to their ability to affect the brain. He wrote, "it is probably not overstating the issue to infer that the nature vs. nurture argument may be simplified to one of DNA or DHA."[13]*

*DNA is the genetic material that is the blueprint for all things in the body. DHA is a long-chain dietary fatty acid called docosahexaenoic acid. It is the most abundant omega-3 fatty acid in the brain and is one of the most important of all fatty acids in the brain.

So, what do the brain-fats actually afford us? The answer lies in the very fabric of the brain's make-up.

THE SEEMING PARADOX OF A BRAIN COMPOSED OF FAT

One of the most remarkable and little-known facts about the human brain is that over sixty percent of its elaborate structure is fat. Using an elegant system of synthesis, conversion, and dietary uptake, the brain weaves a complex tapestry of neural fats to construct one of the most astounding creations in all of nature. The brain is very particular about the kind of fat used in its construction. Like a temple in which each stone is carefully chosen for its purpose, the brain requires specific fats of specific size, length, shape, and function in order to conduct its daily business.

From the retina of your eye to the the nerve centers that control the movement of your arms, brain-fats are required. The nerves that give you the ability to see, hear, smell, touch, and taste require brain-fats. The nerves that allow you to run, jump, throw, play the piano, paint a picture, laugh at a joke, and fall in love all depend upon specific fats. The regions of your brain that govern your mood, behavior, and emotional intelligence require these fats. The regions that give rise to your memory and your ability to learn new things require these fats. In one respect, we are who we are because of fat; not a glamorous notion, but fair.

THE IMPORTANCE OF GOOD CHOICES

Though able to make some of what it needs, the brain is surprisingly dependent upon raw materials from the diet—what we might call brain-fats. With certain fats and at certain ages, the brain has a crucial dependency on dietary sources. In short, if the right fats are not supplied, brain structure is altered. If brain *structure* changes, function changes.

Herein lies the problem and the potential. The average person consuming a traditional Western diet gets nearly forty percent of his or her daily calories from fat. Unfortunately, this abundance has not translated into benefit for the nervous system — quite the opposite. It has been short on the most crucial fats required for the brain.

Over the last one hundred years, the types of fat we consume have changed dramatically. By some estimates, the amount of brain-fats we consume has declined by over eighty percent.[14]

This occurred because many of us switched to animal fats, warm-weather vegetable oils, and processed foods. We once consumed a balance of fat of approximately one to one. Today, scientists estimate the ratio to be as high as thirty to one.[15]

Figure 1
Decreasing Fatty Acid Intake

Changing Fatty Acid Intake: Omega-6:Omega-3 Ratios

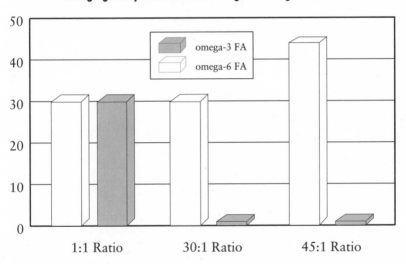

The dietary ratio of omega-6 to omega-3 fatty acids was once approximately 1:1. Modern diets have a ratio of as high as 30:1. The breast milk of some women contains a ratio of as high as 45:1.

The brain's requirement for highly specific fats, coupled with the poor dietary choices of most people living on modern diets, has us on a collision course with ourselves. We now have powerful evidence that millions of people in all walks of life consume a diet of fats that is not at all conducive to building a complex, superbly functioning brain and nervous system. This may be the common feature that underlies a host of behavioral, learning, memory, and neurological disorders, which, up to now, have been considered unrelated. We are beginning to learn that if you want a brain that functions to its full potential and provides a lifetime of vital service, you must pay close attention to dietary fat.

The potential is that with this new knowledge, we may now make precision changes in our diets from very early in life in the hope that we might ensure brain function throughout our lives. We may be able to improve adult function even if dietary fat changes are implemented now. The potential is that we might be able to intervene in a variety of brain disorders by taking advantage of the fact that the brain structure itself might be modified by our fat consumption. We may be able to step beyond current limitations of brain evolution and take our intellectual abilities to new heights.

SHIFTING A PARADIGM: FAT IS NOT ALL BAD

The emerging story of fat and the brain leads us to address a commonly-held misconception: "Isn't fat a bad thing? Aren't we supposed to be cutting out all fat rather than adding fat?" We have become so conditioned by the media to view fat as bad that, for some people, the mere mention of fat conjures images of doom. Grocery stores are filled with low-fat and no-fat foods. Bookstore shelves are lined with books on nearly every health condition telling us how we need to "avoid fat" or "restrict fat." The American Heart Association, through national media campaigns, urges us to dramatically reduce our fat intake.

These ideas are advanced by learned and intelligent people with good training, earnest motives, and sound data to back them up. Now, a book emerges suggesting that fat is necessary for the most complex organ of our bodies — the brain. It may seem inconsistent and confusing, but think about it logically. Fat cannot be simply all bad.

We use fat to make the membranes of cells throughout the body. Even the "dreaded" cholesterol is important. We need cholesterol to make certain hormones, without which our body would become diseased. In fact, cholesterol is absolutely required for your nerve cell membranes. We use fat as fuel to power our cells. We use fat to combat inflammation. We use fat to clot our blood, and to contract and relax our blood vessels. We need fat for proper immune function. Without fat, there would be no skin covering the body to hold the organs in place. Women cannot conceive and bear children if they have an inadequate balance of fats. The list of organs, systems, and biochemical processes in which fat is needed is vast and complex. Without fat none of us would exist.

Does fat contribute to disease? Absolutely. But it is not so simple as just avoiding fat.

A COMMON-SENSE APPROACH TO FAT

Once we've discarded our notion that all fat is bad, we have to establish a new understanding. There are three basic critical points.

- Too much fat in whatever form can lead to disease.
- Too little fat in whatever form can lead to disease.
- The kind of fat and the balance of various fats are the critical features that determine how fat contributes to disease.

We must remember that the brain's major structures have an absolute requirement for fat. Balance of these structural fats appears to be among the important factors that determine your brain's architectural integrity and ultimately, health. This is the point to be emphasized over and over again in this book. You will gain a sense of the balance of fats needed to improve brain function and performance.

WHAT IS FAT? AN INTRODUCTION

Fat is the name given to a broad category of substances we get from our food or make in our bodies. In technical jargon they are referred to as lipids. The family we're most concerned with in this book is called fatty acids. Within the fatty acid family there are saturated, monounsaturated, and polyunsaturated fatty acids. Cholesterol is from another lipid family called sterols.

The brain needs saturated fat, polyunsaturated fat, cholesterol, and a number of other fats. We can make saturated fat with ease. We can make cholesterol with some effort, but we make a lot of it. Polyunsaturated fatty acids are a different matter. Two forms, the essential fatty acids, *must come directly from the diet.* The major brain polyunsaturated fatty acids can be made, but the process can be foiled by many factors (which will be discussed in ensuing chapters). In order to make them, we must get the parent essential fatty acids from the diet. Certain foods do contain brain-fats such as DHA, but many people consume almost none of these foods.

A BRIEF LOOK AT THE BRAIN-FATS AND THE *SMART-FAT* CONCEPT

Brain-fats is a term you'll see occasionally throughout this book. I use the term to refer to dietary fats that are essential to proper brain function. These fatty acids are not found exclusively in the brain, but some are highly concentrated there. Thus, I use the term brain-fats to draw attention to the important role of these fatty acids in the brain. Included are a small number of fatty substances that are found in the brain, which derive from the diet, and which have been studied therapeutically to treat a wide variety of conditions of the nervous system. They have also been used to enhance intellectual function, balance mood, improve learning, and manage stress. Though we cover a range of substances, the brain-fats we'll primarily be discussing are:

> DHA: Docosahexaenoic acid
> AA: Arachidonic acid
> GLA: Gamma-linolenic acid*
> ALA: Alpha-linolenic acid*
> PS: Phosphatidylserine
> PC: Phosphatidylcholine

---

*Not found in brain, but significantly affect the brain by way of its messengers or by formation of brain fats.

DHA will appear repeatedly in this book since it is currently thought to be the most crucial omega-3 fatty acid for the brain found in the diet. Unfortunately, many people get little or no DHA in their diets. Moreover, the parent, alpha-linolenic acid (ALA), from which we can make DHA, is also low in most modern diets.

In later chapters, I describe the *Smart-Fat* concept. While the term brain-fats refers to the actual fats and oils that influence the brain, *Smart-Fat* refers to our *use* of fats and oils. The *Smart-Fat* concept recognizes the wide variety of different fats and oils available in the diet and the brain's reliance upon very select forms. The *Smart-Fat* concept includes:

- The intelligent (*smart*) use of fats and oils.
- Use of specific fats and oils that foster mental, physical, and emotional intelligence (fats that make us *smart*).

When we finish the journey, the importance of DHA and the brain-fats will be clear. The food sources of brain-fats will be clear. In addition to the brain-fats we will look at the brain-fat companions. These are the nutrients needed for defense, energy, and brain-fat formation. We will also explore the harmful fats and oils.

A NEW ERA

For decades, medicine had few certain clues to the origins of heart disease. Once a link was made between dietary fat and heart disease, the approach to this problem was forever transformed.

Similarly, our increasing knowledge of the way in which fat affects the brain may completely transform the way we look at this most vital organ. In fact, this link may turn out to be one of the most important discoveries of the century. We may be on the threshold of a remarkable new era in which we are able to exert profound influence on the structure that determines the very core of our being—the brain itself.

Prepare for a fascinating journey—the story of fatty acids and the brain.

CHAPTER 2

WEAVING THE WEB: THE ROLE OF FAT IN THE BRAIN'S STRUCTURE

At the Olympic Games, a platform diver stood ready, back to the water, toes gripping the platform with heels extended outward. She focused, breathed, paused, and in an instant sprung into the air. Plunging earthward, she guided her body through a series of elegant and sophisticated movements of grand precision. At just the right moment, she emerged from the whirling and spinning to release into the water with hardly a ripple.

Such feats of vision, balance, coordination, reaction, anticipation, and action are astonishing testament to the vast complexity of the human brain and nervous system. To the neuroscientist, these movements are almost incomprehensible in their complexity. The level of neural integration needed to carry out such acts easily dwarfs even the greatest computers on this planet. In short, the human nervous system is one of the most phenomenal wonders in all of nature.

WHERE THE BRAIN-FATS RESIDE

Though highly interdependent, there are many different structures within the brain that make this vast web of complexity function in a coordinated fashion. Observing the brain from above (Figure 2), one would notice nerve fibers that hard-wire one area to another, branches that connect diverse regions, and junctions that allow for communication from one nerve cell to another. Support cells help coordinate a multitude of functions. The nerve membrane (or covering) forms the very basis of the nerve and all its vital activities. Within each nerve are tiny factories that churn out energy for the brain—the most energy-hungry organ in the body.

Figure 2
The Brain from Above

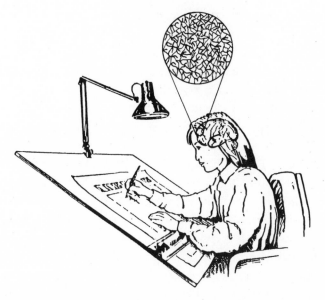

The brain is composed of a complex of billions of cells.

In order for your brain to achieve its optimum level of complexity, and therefore function at its peak, it must receive proper nutrition and proper stimulation at critical points in its development. This begins before conception, persists during gestation, and continues throughout life. Because the brain is predominantly made of fat, almost all of its structures and functions have a crucial dependency upon essential fatty acids, which we get directly from our food.

It may be difficult to comprehend that so complex a structure as the brain is made largely of fat. The very notion conjures images of a white mass curiously adrift inside the skull. However, the brain's fatty composition is not random, but highly specific and elegantly crafted. What follows is a brief description of the precise role of fats in forming the delicate structures that make up your brain and nervous system. With this understanding in place, the profound role of dietary fat in building and maintaining a healthy brain will become evident.

Neurons: The Wiring

Viewing your brain from above, it appears as a grey-white mass of almost gel-like material. Zooming in more closely, we see that this mass is composed of billions of different cells. Some of these are called neurons, the real workhorses of nerve communication. Others, called glial cells, are actually more numerous than neurons and perform an array of vital functions.

Nerve cells are specialized to send information through a vast network to control bodily functions. Some nerves are very long, reaching from the brain to the foot. Others are very short, measuring less than a fraction of an inch. All of them share a common feature; they are surrounded by a covering, or membrane, that is made up of fatty material (Figure 3). Looking more closely at this membrane, we see it is made of a two-layered floating sea of fatty molecules (phospholipids). Zooming closer still, we see the precise location of the fatty acids. From the time the brain is forming to the time of death, essential fatty acids derived from the diet are a critical requirement to make a stable nerve membrane.

Myelin: The Insulating Factor

Surrounding many nerve fibers is a shiny-white substance called myelin. The basic function of myelin is to speed the transmission of nerve impulses; thus, making nerve transmission more efficient and rapid. Myelin is made of various fats, fatty acids, phospholipids, cholesterol, and protein. In fact, about seventy-five percent of myelin comes from fat. Formation of myelin is highly dependent upon nutritional intake because some fatty acids cannot be manufactured by the body. They must be obtained from the diet.

Figure 3
Where Fatty Acids Reside in the Brain

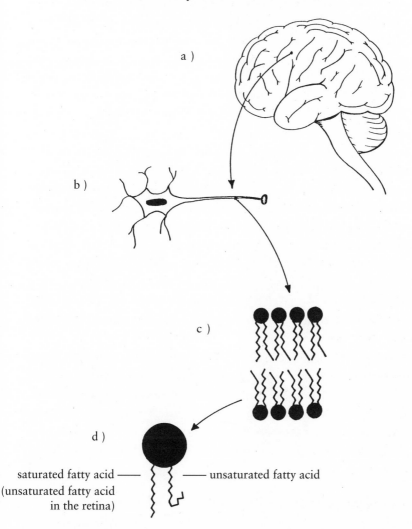

a)

b)

c)

d)

saturated fatty acid ——
(unsaturated fatty acid
in the retina)

—— unsaturated fatty acid

The brain is reduced here into simpler and simpler components eventually revealing the location of the fatty acids. This system is highly organized: a) the brain, b) the nerve cell with a cutaway of the cell membrane, or covering, c) the membrane's two layers, in which the fatty acid "tails" face the interior of the membrane, d) a single phospholipid molecule containing one saturated fat (straight) and one unsaturated fatty acid (curved). In the brain, the unsaturated fatty acid is usually DHA or AA. In the retina, both positions typically contain the unsaturated fatty acid DHA.

If you looked at the myelinated nerve from afar, you would see indents, or nodes, in a regular pattern. These are called nodes of Ranvier, which literally allow the electrical impulse of the nerve to "hop" from node to node. This causes nerve transmission to speed along up to twelve times faster than if the impulse had to trudge its way along the full length of the nerve without such features. The speed of transmission around the body can vary from 1 mile per hour to up to 150 miles per hour. When myelin is damaged, the speed of nerve conduction slows.

Various disease processes lead to destruction of the myelin sheath surrounding nerves. The most well known of these is multiple sclerosis (MS), a disease that strikes adults between age thirty and fifty. Many theories have been put forth regarding the possible cause of multiple sclerosis. As I will discuss later, there are many fatty acid abnormalities in MS, leading us to believe that dietary fat might play a role in the development, prevention, and treatment of this condition.

Myelin formation is also critical to development of the brain in children. There are certain critical windows of development during which nerve fibers must be myelinated. These connections allow the child's brain complexity to unfold and sets the stage for future intelligence. It is now known that if these periods are not met with the right kind of stimulation at the right points in development, nerve connections that have not been made may be pruned or cut out. Likewise, if fatty acids are not provided that ensure efficient myelination of these fibers, the efficiency of brain connections may also be impaired.

Reaching Out: New Brain Growth

One of the remarkable features of the brain is its ability to make new connections based on new experience. Like a tree growing new branches with each new sunset, season, harvest moon, or gust of wind, your brain forms new branches with each encounter of a smiling face, scent from an unfamiliar rose, or musical harmony. As the branches grow in number, so too does the ability of the brain to integrate more complex and diverse functions (Figure 4).

Figure 4
Reaching Out

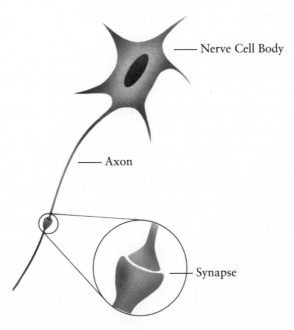

Nerve Cell Body

Axon

Synapse

Nerve cells contain thousands of branches that are used to communicate with other cells. Expansion of the branching network requires structural fatty acids, which are partially dependent upon diet. Through proper diet and stimulation, branching can be encouraged to occur throughout life.

As you learn a new task, more connections are made with different regions of the brain. The brain becomes more fully integrated. As your experiences build, neurons involved with those experiences branch to connect with other sites in the brain, thus associating more of the cortex. This is how we are able to recognize the identity of a familiar voice on the telephone before a name is stated. Our experience with this person has led to formation of many connections in the brain, allowing us to associate the voice with the face, with the name, and with many things about the individual.

Like a growing tree, any time a nerve cell makes a new branch it requires new raw materials. Fatty acids make up a large percentage of the nerve membrane itself as well as the myelin sheath that surrounds it. With proper fatty acids available branching can flourish. If brain-fats are not available in needed amounts, branching may suffer.

Making Connections

One of the most critical features of the human brain is the ability of the neuron branches to make connections with other neurons. These connections are called synapses, or the places where one nerve cell connects with another. At this junction between cells is a space, or gap, called the synaptic cleft. This area is much like the gap in a spark plug. Chemical messengers are released from the synaptic bulb into the gap and diffuse through the space until they meet the surface of the other neuron. Once the messenger interacts with the proper "receiver," or receptor, on the other side, the nerve begins firing.

In its lifetime, a single neuron may make perhaps 6,000 to 20,000 synaptic connections with other neurons located in various portions of the brain. The synapse is where the real business of nerve communication and brain activity takes place. The number of synapses made by a nerve has a greater bearing on intelligence and brain performance than the number of nerve cells.

Here again, fatty acids, or brain-fats, are critical. The delicate membrane of the synapse has an extremely high concentration of long-chain fatty acids.[1] In fact, the synapse has a higher concentration of the brain-fat DHA than almost any tissue in the body. If these requirements are not met, neurons do not fire with normal efficiency. Problems can develop in the neuron, leading to poor function or even neuron death.

Sending the Signal

In order for areas of the brain to communicate with one another, substances called neurotransmitters are released. Neurotransmitters are usually proteins or amino acids that are released by one nerve, then drift across the synapse to interact with the next nerve on the information highway of the brain.

For example, the neurotransmitter serotonin is crucial to normal mood and behavior. When serotonin function is altered,

Figure 5
Making Connections

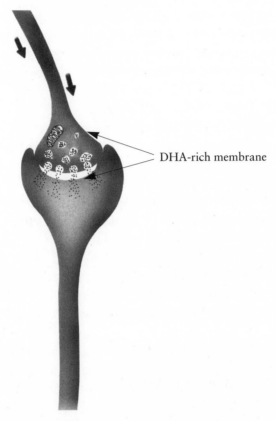

DHA-rich membrane

A single nerve may make up to 20,000 connections with other cells. The place where these cells connect is called the synapse. The portion of the nerve making the connection is called the synaptic membrane. This part of the nerve has a higher concentration of the brain-fat DHA than almost any tissue in the body.

mood changes like depression can occur. Some of the most popular prescription drugs on the market (e.g. Prozac) are designed to modify the serotonin system. While the neurotransmitters like serotonin are themselves not fats, their ability to land in the right spot and trigger their action may significantly depend upon fatty acids. In this way, fatty acids have a profound affect on the efficiency of the neurotransmitter system.

Docking the Ship

Neurotransmitters all have a specific shape based on their structure. As they swirl around in the sea of fluid near the nerve cell synapse they are drawn to structures on the nerve cell surface called receptors. The receptors are also very specific in their shape. They are designed to accommodate a particular neurotransmitter, fitting together like a lock and key.

Another way to view this relationship is like a ship and a dock. The neurotransmitter is like the ship, while the receptor is like a dock. The ship (neurotransmitter) carries the cargo (information). Once it docks (with the receptor), the cargo can be unloaded and the information sent to the appropriate place.

Each receptor is held in place in the cell membrane by molecules called phospholipids and fatty acids. Much like our analogy above, the fatty acids might be likened to the poles holding the dock in place. If the poles are not placed properly the dock may drift or change the shape of its opening. When this occurs, the ship may no longer fit. It cannot dock and, therefore, cannot unload its cargo.

In the nervous system, if the "ship" cannot dock, the nerve signal is not sent. Nerve communication changes. In essence, you short-circuit the communication of the nerve. We now have strong evidence that specific fatty acids have a strong influence on the "docking" of neurotransmitters with their receptors.[2] Improving fatty acid status can improve the action of serotonin, insulin, dopamine, and other neurotransmitters. Fatty acid supplements have even been shown to improve the action of antidepressant drugs. Thus, dietary fat can influence this very important aspect of nerve communication and potentially influence mood, behavior, learning, and even our ability to move our bodies.

SEEING WITH CLARITY: FATTY ACIDS AND VISION

Receptors in your retina that allow you to see are marvelously specialized to receive light and quickly translate that information into diverse signals. These impulses are then sent to regions of the

Figure 6
Docking the Ship

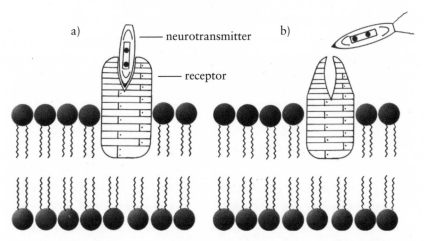

a) —— neurotransmitter   b)

—— receptor

Nerve cells communicate by releasing neurotransmitters into the synaptic space. While in this space, the neurotransmitter molecules seek a "port," or receptor, into which they neatly fit. The ability to "dock" depends upon the shape of both the neurotransmitter and the receptor. Fatty acid balance affects the shape of the dock (receptor), which may make it difficult for the neurotransmitter (ship) to fit. This may slow nerve communication and affect many aspects of brain function. Part a) shows the proper "fit" of the ship in the dock. Part b) illustrates how changing the dock's shape prevents the ship from docking.

brain to interpret them and give them life. The portion of your retina called the photoreceptor is lined with a membrane, or covering, even more specialized than normal nerves. This delicate fatty membrane uses DHA (docosahexaenoic acid) to conduct its rapid work. In fact, the retina has the highest concentrations of this fatty acid of any tissue in the body.[3]

The fatty acid DHA is crucial for formation of the retina in the fetus and infant. Studies conducted over the past five years suggest that infants who received adequate fatty acids such as DHA have better visual acuity and image processing than those not receiving adequate DHA.[4] It is therefore necessary for proper visual function.

While important in children, there is evidence that a constant supply of DHA may be needed throughout life in order to preserve vision. This comes from knowledge that the retina's photoreceptor cells are shed daily and replaced with new cells. In order to retain vital visual capacity, DHA must be provided to the newly forming cells. Commenting on the need for DHA in vision, Dr. Artemis Simopoulos, of the Center for Genetics, Nutrition, and Health in New York, suggests that "[DHA] is important in the function of photoreceptors [of the retina] and might even improve visual function in the aged."[5]

SMELL AND THE EMOTIONAL BRAIN

One of the most primitive parts of the brain is our olfactory system, giving us our sense of smell. These nerves take in molecules wafting about in the air and identify them with awesome precision. This process is directly linked to our emotional brain and dramatically affects our behavior. For example, a baby can identify its mother entirely by smell. Odors can trigger recall of profoundly wonderful memories or tragic encounters based on the odor with which the original event is associated.

Olfactory nerves are the only part of the nervous system directly exposed to the outside world. They are among the shortest nerves in the body and have the quickest route to the brain's core. Unlike other senses like vision, olfactory neurons go directly to primitive areas of the brain's cortex, bypassing a central processing area called the thalamus.

There are so many parts of the brain that receive olfactory connections that listing those parts of the brain that do not receive them is easier than listing those that do. Among other things, the olfactory arrangement gives an unusually and widespread influence on the parts of the brain that have roles in emotion, motivation, reproduction, feeding, conscious perception, and certain kinds of memory.

Olfactory receptors continually grow, die, and regenerate, in a cycle that lasts about four to eight weeks. These olfactory receptor cells are the only *neurons* in the nervous system that are regularly replaced throughout life.[6] The structure of these nerves is dependent, in part, on fatty acids. Each cycle of reproduction of olfactory nerves demands appropriate fatty acids. Because they are exposed to the outside world, their fatty layer is susceptible to damage from cigarette smoke, air pollution, toxic fumes, or trauma. Many people who have lost their sense of smell have significant changes in their behavior and ability to interpret the world.

Because neurons of the olfactory system are dependent upon the integrity of the fatty membrane and because the olfactory system so strongly affects emotion, the brain-fats may affect our moods, emotions, and ability to understand our world by virtue of their effect on smell and the limbic system.

FATS, OILS, AND YOUR BODY CELLS

All of the complex features that make our brains remarkable are only possible if the makeup of the brain follows its intended pattern. This pattern requires particular fatty acids and other nutrients throughout life. This book is about the dramatic ways in which the fats and oils you put in your mouth affect the brain. But we should not forget that your entire body is made up of cells that require fat for their basic structure.

Your body is made up of cells, each of which has a covering made up of various substances. One of the most important substances forming the basic structure is fatty acids. If we took every cell of your body, opened them up, and laid their membranes out flat, they would cover an area roughly the size of ten football fields. Imagine, you are perhaps five- to six-feet tall and the surface area of your cell coverings span the size of a football stadium parking lot.[7] If you could view this from the air it would probably look like a thin layer of oil spread out over a vast distance.

This oil-slick derived from your cell membranes would consist of fat molecules from the salad oil, mayonnaise, seeds, nuts, butter, lard, steak, fish, french fries, potato chips, and other fatty parts of the food you have eaten over the past days to weeks to months. Some of the oils might contribute to membranes of high integrity, while others are not at all desirable for peak cell membrane structure. In essence, the actual structure of your cells, the stones of the palace, are based on what you put in your mouth.

Like the brain, your other cells are very specific about the fats and oils they use for their construction. If you vary the balance of fats too far in one direction or another, the makeup of your cells changes. For most of your cell membranes, the fatty acids must come directly from the oils in your diet. You cannot make them.

In this chapter, we have explored the important role that fatty acids play in forming the *structure* of the brain. But the brain fats play another, equally crucial role, which affects *function* of the brain in dramatic ways. That is, as messengers.

CHAPTER 3

KEEPING YOUR BRAIN IN THE FLOW: THE MESSENGERS

Beyond their important role in building the *structure* of nerves and, thus, the brain itself, fatty acids have another crucial role—as messengers. These messengers become the signalers of activity throughout the body. They tell the immune cells whether to wake up or settle down. They tell the blood vessels whether to narrow or widen. The messengers tell the blood platelets whether to stick together or separate, thus affecting the clotting of blood. The messengers regulate inflammation. For every messenger that performs one function, there is another that performs the opposite function. In a sense, the messengers are like a town crier, signaling a call to action or signaling that all is well.

These messengers come under a variety of technical names, but each of them has something in common: they are made from essential fatty acids that come from your diet. Some messengers are formed from omega-6 fatty acids, while others are formed from omega-3 fatty acids. In many cases, the messengers that are formed from omega-6 fatty acids perform the opposite function of those formed from omega-3 fatty acids.

BUILDING THE MESSENGERS: FROM DIETARY FAT TO PROSTAGLANDINS

The membranes of your nerves, blood cells, and blood vessels are made of trillions of fatty acid molecules. The balance of these fatty acids within the membranes is determined largely by your diet. When your diet is balanced in omega-6 and omega-3 fatty acids, your cells are balanced in these fatty acids as well. When your diet has too little omega-3 fatty acids your cell membranes have too little omega-3 fatty acids.

✓   Fatty acids that form the structure of your cell membranes become messengers when a call to action is sent out. This call can be in the form of trauma, a virus, a bacteria, a free radical, a toxic chemical, a heavy metal, or some other trigger. Once the call to action has been sent, your cell's fatty acids are released from the membrane and are chemically transformed into highly active hormonelike substances. Once the hormonelike messengers are released they exert powerful and profound effects on a vast array of functions within the brain.

These messengers are given the name prostaglandins because they were originally discovered in the prostate gland. Now we know that prostaglandins are produced throughout the body. Prostaglandins (PG) are formed directly through a series of steps from dietary fatty acids. Those we're concerned with are called PGE1, PGE2, and PGE3.

PGE1 is formed from dietary linoleic acid. This is the fatty acid predominant in corn oil, sunflower oil, sesame oil, and safflower oil. PGE2 is formed from the fatty acid arachidonic acid. This fatty acid is found only rarely in plants and is most common in animal meat. PGE3 is formed from the fatty acid EPA (eicosapentaenoic acid), found in salmon, mackerel, herring, sardines, and other fish. Another form of PG3 is formed from the fatty acid DHA (docosahexaenoic acid).

PGE1 is important in the nervous system as it affects the release of compounds from nerve cells that transmit nerve impulses. It tends to have anti-inflammatory properties and is immune-enhancing. It can reduce fluid accumulation and has a significant effect on the nervous system. Some doctors have manipulated the PGE1 pathway to improve depression, multiple sclerosis, PMS- (premenstrual syndrome) related mood changes, schizophrenia, ADHD (attention deficit hyperactivity disorder), and other conditions.

Figure 7
How the Brain Messengers Are Formed from Fatty Acids

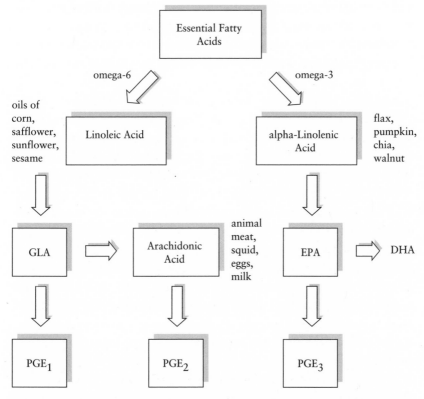

Dietary fatty acids are converted into compounds called prostaglandins, leukotrienes, thromboxane, and prostacyclin, which have a tremendous effect on the brain's blood flow. They also affect the brain's immune system and the neurotransmitter system. (Prostaglandins PGE1, 2, 3.)

✔ PGE2 is a highly inflammatory substance. It can cause swelling, increased pain sensitivity, and increased blood viscosity. Some of the other compounds associated with PGE2 can cause blood platelet clumping, spasm of blood vessels, and accumulation of inflammatory cells in an area, and over the long term can change the way in which nerve cells communicate. These compounds can also cause an overactive immune system within the nervous system, chiding the immune cells to attack the host. Elevated PGE2 has been found in a number of problems affecting mood, behavior, and nervous system function.

Substances called leukotrienes are related to PGE2 in that they are made from the fatty acid arachidonic acid. However, leukotrienes are even more potent inflammatory substances. They have been estimated to be 1,000 to 10,000 times more inflammatory than histamine, the substance associated with the runny nose and watery eyes of allergy and hay fever. They signal white blood cells to travel to an area. This is good when you need them, but white cells can do a lot of damage when present in excess.

The PGE2 family is sometime viewed as a "bad guy" because of the powerful inflammatory potential it possesses. In reality, we need this family for many vital functions. The problem arises when the system is out of balance, when there is too much activity in this family. This balance is tied to fatty acid balance.

PGE3 tends to be mildly anti-inflammatory and immune enhancing. It is thought to counter the affects of the powerfully inflammatory PGE2 substances. It prevents blood platelets from clumping and helps prevent blood vessel spasm. Fatty acids important in PGE3 formation, like EPA and DHA, can also reduce arachidonic acid in the cells. This reduces the chance of producing messengers from arachidonic acid and is one way that these fatty acids can alter the production of highly inflammatory messengers.

Food Sources of EFA and Their Messengers

PG Series	Fatty Acid	Fatty Acid Family	Food Sources
1	Linoleic	n-6	Sunflower, safflower, sesame, corn
1	gamma-Linolenic	n-6	Primrose, borage, and black currant seed oil
2	Arachidonic	n-6	Animal meat, milk, eggs, squid, warm-water fish
3	alpha-Linolenic	n-3	Flax, canola, pumpkin, chia, walnut
3	EPA	n-3	Cold water fish, algae (some)
3	DHA	n-3	Cold water fish, algae (some)

MESSENGERS OUT OF BALANCE

This messenger system is necessary to control a remarkable array of functions within the body and the brain. It is generally able to do so as long as the fatty acid *balance* is appropriate. Should one family of fatty acids be present in greater amounts than another, the scales are tipped toward the fatty acid type that predominates. The most common scenario of imbalance is that relating to arachidonic acid and the PGE2 pathway.

For example, if you consume a diet high in arachidonic acid, this fatty acid becomes predominant in your cell membranes. When an event happens in the body that might trigger inflammation, the inflammatory portion, of which arachidonic acid is a part, works very effectively. However, once its work is done and the process needs to be subdued, there may not be an adequate balance of other fatty acid messengers to do the job. In one sense, the cells are "primed for inflammation" with inadequate messengers to properly shut off the system.

Messengers in the arachidonic acid pathway come under the names PGE2, thromboxane, and leukotriene. All are powerfully active and can significantly alter brain activity when present in excess. Unfortunately, the typical Western diet is one that favors the arachidonic acid messengers. Occasionally, arachidonic acid levels are too low. This also effects brain function and requires a specific strategy to balance fats and oils.

We recently measured the blood cells of a young boy who had developmental delays, attention deficit, and hyperactivity. The level of arachidonic acid in his cells was almost fifty percent above normal. In one sense, his cells were primed to form the most inflammatory of the brain messengers. I believe his brain is not functioning efficiently because of the broad effects of the arachidonic acid messengers.

He has been on a diet that improved his omega-3 fatty acid intake and restricted food sources of arachidonic acid. Supplemental doses of the fatty acids ALA (alpha-linolenic acid), DHA, and GLA (gamma-linolenic acid) are a part of this program. We also had him avoid factors that disrupt the fatty acid pathways and began him on nutrients that will help balance his fatty acid pathways. This is only one phase of his program, but his early response has been very encouraging. His teachers, parents, and grandparents have all noticed improvement in his concentration, mood, ability to cooperate, and ability to take his own initiative. His fine and gross motor functions have improved and he is doing better in physical activity.

Leo Galland, M.D., of New York, notes that using nutritional strategies that modify the messengers has shown profound results in conditions such as multiple sclerosis, depression, premenstrual depression, attention deficit, hyperactivity, and schizophrenia.

Galland has observed that giving essential fatty acids to a patient with these conditions can have a profound effect on their recovery. He uses attention deficit hyperactivity as an example where giving fatty acids is likely to affect the messenger activity. Dr. Galland states that some children with attention deficit hyperactivity respond to the fatty acid GLA found in primrose oil, while others with the same condition may respond better to ALA found in flax oil. This difference in responses, he reflects, may be due not only to the structural effects of the fatty acids, but to the messenger effects on the brain.[1]

Messengers and Mood: The Story of Megan

Megan was a bright woman who had been near the top of her class in both high school and college. She was emotionally healthy, had a wonderful family, and by all accounts was very stable. However, during the premenstrual period her mood shifted dramatically. She became weepy, felt hopeless, shouted angrily, and became depressed. The principal in a small business, she was used to being on top and getting things done. The despair and disruption she experienced during these times made living her life an arduous task.

Megan began taking six evening primrose oil perles daily. This is a source of the fatty acid GLA, which we will discuss in the next chapter. GLA is not found in the brain. However, it has been used frequently in medicine to balance the inflammatory and anti-inflammatory messengers that influence the brain. I believe the improvement in Megan's mood was related to the effect GLA has on increasing the messenger PGE1 and decreasing PGE2.

David Perlmutter, M.D., a neurologist from Naples, Florida, has found that using essential fatty acids to modify the messengers can be enormously helpful in certain disorders of the brain. He believes that it is necessary to balance the messengers using fatty acids like GLA, while also providing specific omega-3 fatty acids to build brain membranes. Dr. Perlmutter now considers this approach a focal point of treating his patients with multiple sclerosis.[2] He believes that by reducing saturated fat, increasing GLA, and increasing omega-3 fatty acids such as ALA and DHA one can strongly influence the messengers and reduce the adverse effects of the inflammatory messengers.

Alcohol can also disrupt the messengers. This may be one reason for the hangover associated with consumption of alcohol and may also account for some of the mood and cognitive changes. When specific fatty acids such as GLA and DHA are used, one can encourage the body to produce the proper messengers that will maintain brain function. Some of the most powerful and potent messengers with regard to brain power are those that affect the brain's blood supply.

PRESERVING THE FLOW:
MESSENGERS AND THE BRAIN'S BLOOD SUPPLY

Despite its relatively small size, only two percent of total body weight, your adult brain uses a tremendous twenty-five percent of the oxygen consumed by your entire body. In the developing fetus, the brain uses seventy percent of the energy provided by the mother. During the first year of life, the brain continues to use sixty percent of the energy generated by the child's body.

In order to maintain the delivery of such vast amounts of energy-supporting products to the brain, it must command nearly twenty percent of the heart's output. Imagine, almost one-fifth of your heart's activity is in service to the brain. Consider also that the brain receives an amazing twenty-five times more blood than the equivalent weight of tissue in a resting arm or leg.[3] This requires a complex network of vessels and an efficiently working heart.

Hitting a tennis ball, memorizing your neighbor's phone number, or finding your way to the grocery store are all dependent upon blood flow to the brain. Performing well in school, taking an exam, or getting the job done at work all require efficient blood flow to the brain. Even your mood, emotions, and behavior are dependent upon blood supply. Any restriction in the supply weakens brain function. There are no exceptions.

THE BRAIN'S BLOOD SUPPLY THROUGHOUT YOUR LIFETIME

The blood supply and the brain are so closely intertwined that they develop simultaneously. The fate of the brain is at all times tied directly to the developing blood supply. If there is interruption of the blood supply during a critical fetal period, the corresponding portion of the brain may be negatively affected. In an adult, the gradual loss of blood supply to the brain can impair mental function that creeps up slowly over time.

Scientists are beginning to learn that dietary factors may cause the blood vessels to begin narrowing very early in life. For example, when doctors studied the blood vessels of children ranging from age one to fifteen they discovered that the vessels already showed evidence of narrowing. Narrowed blood vessels were even found in the youngest children studied.[4]

When the arteries of such children were analyzed for fatty acid composition two striking findings stood out. The blood vessels were too low in omega-3 fatty acids (EPA) and too high in omega-6 fatty acids (linoleic acid).[5] This is similar to another study of children aged three to eighteen years in which doctors studied the fatty acids of blood. They learned that there was a significant reduction in omega-3 fatty acids and too much omega-6 linoleic acid.[6]

All of this brings us to one important conclusion: From very early in life, your dietary fats have a profound effect on the vessels that supply vital oxygen and nutrients to the brain. Many people today consume a diet imbalanced in fats that are crucial to maintaining a healthy blood supply. Because of this, early in life the blood vessels begin narrowing and will influence brain function throughout the lifespan.

Of course, declining blood supply to the brain because of vessel narrowing is not an inevitable fate. Its close correlation to our intake of the proper fats and oils gives us the opportunity to set the stage early in life for optimum brain function. Even if you intervene later in life, you have the ability to make meaningful changes and preserve brain function.

WHEN CHARLIE GOT LOST

Charlie was a successful businessman in his fifties whose real passion was singing. He had a beautiful voice and was regularly invited to sing at church services, weddings, and other gatherings. One summer afternoon, Charlie was preparing offstage to give a performance. A friend strolled into the backstage area and found Charlie slumped over on a chair with his head in his hand.

"Charlie, are you OK?" queried his friend Allen.

"Where am I?" he muttered. "What am I doing here?"

"You mean you don't know? You're here to sing at the wedding."

"What wedding?" the confused Charlie responded.

Normally quick-witted and socially astute, Charlie was at a complete loss as to his surroundings and his purpose for being there. He was terribly frightened. Within a few hours, however, Charlie gradually regained his awareness of who he was and why he was at the gathering. He had experienced a *transient ischemic attack* (TIA)—brief period of time where blood flow to the brain is reduced. The symptoms are determined by the area of the brain that has been briefly deprived of its blood supply. In a TIA, the blood flow usually returns and an individual regains function. But it is a sign that something is slowing blood flow and must be addressed. It can be a prelude to a stroke.

Charlie was fortunate that his blood supply returned along with his mental faculties. Loss of these faculties is something adults fear most as they mature. But as noted above, changes in blood supply to the brain can occur at any age and are strongly influenced by dietary fats and oils.

HOW FATS AND OILS AFFECT THE BRAIN'S BLOOD SUPPLY

There are at least four ways that fat affects the brain's blood supply. First, the essential fatty acids that make up the membranes of your nerves also make up the membranes of the blood vessels. Though the actual fatty acids are slightly different, the need for omega-6 and omega-3 balance is still important. Fatty acid imbalance can set the stage for poor structural tone of the vessel walls.

Second, the same essential fatty acids affect the formation of messengers that influence blood vessel spasm. When you consume the right balance of fatty acids, chemicals (called prostacyclins) are produced that tend to relax blood vessels. This is desirable if you want to maintain oxygen flow to the brain. In this way, the messengers help prevent constricting of blood vessels and maintain a rich supply of oxygen to the brain.

The third way in which fats affect the brain's blood supply is by changing the blood viscosity, or thickness. While blood seems watery, it is rich with millions of molecules and cells. Blood becomes thicker, or sludge-like, when some of the formed elements stick together. The factors that stick together are called platelets, tiny little microscopic cells that drift in the sea of blood. When arachidonic acid gets too high, its products (thromboxanes) can signal the blood platelets to clump when you don't want them to clump. This can influence blood flow to the brain. Anything that might cause the blood to thicken interferes with the delivery of needed oxygen, nutrients, and raw materials to a site.

The Causes of Blood Sludging: When the Wrong Fats Are Too High

Another factor also causes blood sludging (though it is not a messenger function), impairing vital oxygen delivery to the brain. When certain blood-fats get too high they make the blood thicker. The higher the fat level, the thicker the blood. As blood gets thicker it may slow oxygen to the brain and affect its function.

The result may be changes in mood and behavior. The typical fats involved in making the blood more viscous are triglycerides and cholesterol.

In a landmark study published in 1994, Dr. Charles Glueck discovered that elevated triglycerides, high total cholesterol, and low HDL (or "good") cholesterol were the sole cause of depression in patients being treated for a familial form of hyperlipidemia.[7] In an interview in *Psychology Today*, he stated, "We have shown that in patients with high triglycerides who were in a depressive state, the more you lower the triglycerides, the more you alleviate the depression."[8] Other investigators have found that modifying blood fats can influence hostility, aggression, a domineering attitude, and other aspects of mood.[9]

This work suggests that when brain function seemed to be affected we should investigate factors that alter the brain's blood supply. This may involve, among other things, looking at blood-fat levels as well as the dietary balance of omega-6 and omega-3 fatty acids.

Five Steps to Preserving the Flow*

1. Keep triglycerides between 40 and 170.
2. Keep total cholesterol between 160 and 200.
3. Raise HDL cholesterol above 35.
4. Keep omega-3 fatty acid intake adequate.
5. Consume modest saturated fat and keep total fat between 20 and 30 percent.

THE BRAIN'S IMMUNE SYSTEM

In addition to nerve cells, the brain contains another family of cells called glial cells. One of these, the microglia, is part of the brain's immune system. Microglia, when "switched on" can,

---

*There are, or course, other factors that influence blood supply to the brain. Important among these is elevated blood homocysteine. However, the focus of this book is to show the influence of fats and oils on the brain.

under some circumstances, attack and destroy existing nerve cells in the brain. The signals that tell the microglia to wake up are sent by chemicals called cytokines. The balance and regulation of the brain's immune system is very complex, but the cytokines are strongly influenced by essential fatty acid balance.[10] In fact, we'll see later that fatty acid balance may even effect tumors of the brain that involve glial cells. Thus, by maintaining the right balance of fats and oils you may be able to maintain balance within your brain's immune system.

THE DUAL ROLE OF FATS IN THE BRAIN

In the previous chapters, we learned that specific fatty acids are needed to form the actual membrane, or covering of the nerves. In this way, the brain fats have an important role in forming the brain *structure*. Now we learn that fats have an additional effect on the brain by their powerful influence on the brain's messengers and thus, on the brain's blood supply.

The fatty acids that affect brain structure are, surprisingly, some of the same fatty acids that affect your brain's blood vessel function. Because of this dual effect, getting optimal fats and oils very early in life is crucial to maintaining peak brain function. It is also necessary to prevent many of the problems of deteriorating brain health so common as we age.

In the next chapter, we'll explore the specific fats and oils in more depth.

PART II

FINDING THE RIGHT FATS AND OILS

CHAPTER 4

SMART FATS AND OILS: THE FATS THAT FORM THE BRAIN

As we more deeply understand the powerful effect of fat on the brain, we are drawn to contemplate one of the most peculiar developments of modern culture. All across America, hospitals have opened fast food establishments within their walls. Not only is this a growing reality, but the hospitals are actually quite proud of such alliances. I must say, watching physicians and patients carrying burgers, fries, and deep-fried chicken nuggets down the halls of one of our nation's prestigious medical teaching institutions, leaves me with a feeling of irony.

In many ways, this reflects our cultural values surrounding food and nutrition. As the story of fat and the brain continues to unfold throughout this book, we will see that our cultural marriage to the quick, easy, high-fat lifestyle may come with an enormous price. Doctors have tried for decades to get people to change their diets in an effort to prevent heart disease. However, to most people, heart disease is a distant consequence that usually happens to someone else. Knowledge that the brain is made of fat and that our habits might affect everything from our mood to our children's behavior, makes the consequence more immediate and tangible.

To bring this concept closer into the realm of everyday life, it is helpful to understand more about the fats and oils, their origins, and their relationships. This begins with understanding the family tree of essential fatty acids (EFA).

UNDERSTANDING FATS AND OILS: THE FAMILY TREE

Most fats are derived from animal or vegetable food sources. All of the fats share a common feature in that they are made of carbon and hydrogen with a molecule or two of oxygen. What separates the common fats is the number of carbon atoms and the way in which these atoms are arranged. There are two main categories of fatty acids in the diet that we'll discuss: saturated and unsaturated. When all the carbon atoms in the chain are linked to hydrogen atoms at all possible positions, the fatty acid is considered to be *saturated,* or filled, with hydrogen. If two carbon atoms are double bonded to each other, each has one less hydrogen and the fatty acid is considered *unsaturated.*

Figure 8
Saturated and Unsaturated Fatty Acids

Saturated Fatty Acid

C-C-C-C-C-C-C-C-C-C-C-C-C-C-C-C-C

Monounsaturated Fatty Acid

C-C-C-C-C-C-C-C-C=C-C-C-C-C-C-C-C

Polyunsaturated Fatty Acid

C-C-C-C-C-C=C-C-C=C-C-C-C-C-C-C-C

Saturated fatty acids contain single bonds (-)between all carbon atoms (C). Monounsaturated have one position where there is a double bond (=) between carbons. Polyunsaturated fatty acids have more than one position with double bonds. Each double bond added to a fatty acid causes a "bend" or "kink" in the molecule. (These are shown without "bends" for simplicity.) The most highly unsaturated fatty acids like DHA, have as many as six double bonds and are U-shaped.

If the fatty acid has only one double bond it is said to be mo-nounsaturated. If it has two or more double bonds it is said to be polyunsaturated. This feature of double bonds dramatically affects the properties of the fats and oils. As the number of double bonds increases in a fatty acid, the shape, electrical properties, and value to the brain increase significantly. In fact, one of the brain's principal fatty acids, DHA, contains six double bonds. It appears that no other fatty acid can provide the unique properties that DHA gives to the brain. Increasing double bonds also means the fatty acid is more susceptible to rancidity. This characteristic of the brain's fatty acids will be explored in Chapter Six.

Fats in food are mixtures of saturated and unsaturated fatty acids. In general, fats containing saturated fatty acids are solid at room temperature. Included are the fats of animal products such as beef, lamb, pork, suet, lard, and some dairy products. Fats that contain mostly unsaturated fatty acids are usually liquid at room temperature and are commonly referred to as oils. Oils are mostly from plant sources such as flax, sesame, sunflower, walnut, algae, and soybean. However, some fish, squid, and other sea creatures contain high amounts of unsaturated fatty acids.

The Essential Fatty Acids

Essential means that our bodies cannot make the substance and must get it directly from the diet. In the world of fatty acids two are considered essential. They are called **linoleic** acid (LA) and *alpha*-**linolenic** acid (ALA). Linoleic acid is an omega-6 fatty acid that is commonly found in foods such as the oils of sunflower, safflower, corn, and sesame. Alpha-linolenic acid is an omega-3 fatty acid that is found in foods such as the oils of flax and walnut, and green leafy vegetables. The human body is unable to make linoleic acid from alpha-linolenic acid and vice versa. Therefore, we must have them both.

It is from these essential fatty acids that our bodies make the vital brain-fats and the vital messengers that help regulate a vast array of body activity. Without the essential fatty acids, our bodies run out of the building blocks our cells require to maintain peak function.

Fatty acids used by the brain, what we can call brain-fats or neural fatty acids, contain both saturated and unsaturated forms. The key difference: saturated fatty acids can be easily made by the body from simple raw materials. In the brain, nearly one third of the fatty acids are polyunsaturated. These fatty acids are derived directly from the diet.[1] In the brain, there is little linoleic or alpha-linolenic acid. The brain prefers arachidonic acid (AA) and docosahexaenoic acid (DHA). For the brain, these two fatty acids might be considered essential.

Understanding the Omega Factor

Scientists divide unsaturated fatty acids into several categories based on the position of the first double bond, or kink in the fatty acid molecule. For our purposes, you must know only omega-9, omega-6 and omega-3. Omega-6 fatty acids have their first double bond at the sixth carbon from the end. Omega-3 fatty acids have their first double bond at the third carbon from the end. Functionally, this makes them very different. The designation **n-6** is often used to denote omega-6, and **n-3** is used to denote omega-3.

The major omega-9, omega-6, and omega-3 fatty acids are listed below. In each case, the fatty acids are listed in order of their formation from the parent essential fatty acid. (See glossary for explanation of the scientific designation.) The fatty acids found in the brain are listed with an asterisk(*).

Omega-9 Fatty Acids	**Scientific Designation**
Oleic acid	18:1n-9
Omega-6 Fatty Acids	
Linoleic acid (LA)	18:2n-6
gamma-linolenic acid (GLA)	18:3n-6
Arachidonic acid (AA)*	20:4n-6
Omega-3 Fatty Acids	
alpha-linolenic acid (ALA)	18:3n-3
Eicosapentaenoic acid (EPA)	20:5n-3
Docosahexaenoic acid (DHA)*	22:6n-3

SHIFTING THE BALANCE OF BRAIN-FATS

A key to understanding why fatty acids are so important to the brain is to know one basic concept: Balance. If one family of fatty acids is present in too great an amount the balance of power is shifted to the activity of that family. In fact, the two essential fatty acids, LA and ALA, compete for the same enzymes. If LA predominates in the diet, it commands most of the enzymes. If ALA predominates, it commands a greater share.

The n-6:n-3 Ratio

Since dietary balance of fatty acids is so important, we talk about ratios, comparing one item to another. It has been estimated that, years ago, our diets contained omega-6 and omega-3 fatty acids in about a one-to-one ratio (1:1). For every one gram of omega-6 oils there was one gram of omega-3 oils. Scientists believe this was ideal for human brain function.

Today, the ratio is estimated to be from 20 to 30:1.[2] This means that there are thirty parts omega-6 fatty acids for every one part of omega-3 fatty acids. In mother's breast milk the ratio is sometimes even worse—as high as 45:1. Infant formula commonly had a ratio of about 10:1, but up until 1997 none of this was in the form of DHA.[3,4]

This changing ratio of fatty acids appears to have significant implications for brain function. This becomes our starting point as we explore ways to foster peak brain performance by balancing dietary fats and oils.

HOW WE GOT WHERE WE ARE

Dr. Donald Rudin, author of *The Omega-3 Phenomenon*, has estimated that, over the past seventy-five years, we have reduced our omega-3 fatty acid consumption by eighty percent.[5] He cites the following reasons for this significant decline in one of our most vital brain nutrient families:[6]

- Increased consumption of omega-3-deficient warm weather oils (corn, sunflower, sesame, etc.)
- Hydrogenation of oils in commercial processing
- Decreased fish consumption
- Loss of cereal germ (which contains the fatty acids) by modern milling practices
- 2500% increase in trans fatty acid intake (which interferes with fatty acid synthesis)
- 250% increase in sugar intake (which interferes with the enzymes of fatty acid synthesis)

In an article in the *Journal of Orthomolecular Medicine,* Dr. Rudin states, "Studies show that most of these nutritional deviations interfere synergistically with EFA utilization, thus effectively increasing EFA requirement, even as omega-3 fatty acid availability declines. Consequently, the *effective* omega-3 fatty acid equivalent deficiency is greatly in excess of the 80 percent dietary depletion." In essence, Rudin suggests that the above factors have an additive effect that make the practical fatty acid deficiency even greater.[7]

It is my hope that we can take the revelations of Dr. Rudin and make changes to our dietary practices that bring them more in line with our body's needs. This begins with understanding a bit more about the two principal brain fatty acids: DHA and AA. This is followed by an exploration of the other fatty acids that influence the brain's messengers.

DHA: THE CRITICAL LONG-CHAIN FATTY ACID FOR THE BRAIN

For many years, we knew little about DHA other than the fact that it accompanied the fatty acid EPA in various kinds of fish. Over the past two decades we have learned that DHA is the critical long-chain omega-3 fatty acid found in the brain. Our bodies have the ability to make DHA from the essential fatty acid ALA, but this process is often very inefficient. Thus, we seem to have a requirement for preformed DHA in the diet that cannot be met by other fatty acids. In this way, DHA may be a conditionally-essential fatty acid and essential for the brain.

DHA is concentrated in parts of the brain that require a high degree of electrical activity. This includes the synaptosome, where one nerve ending communicates with another. DHA is heavily concentrated in the photoreceptor of the retina and is vital for proper vision. DHA is also found in high amounts in the mitochondria of nerve cells. These are the tiny bodies that generate all of the energy that gives the brain life.[8] All organs of the body are exposed to DHA as it circulates through the bloodstream, but the requirement of the brain is so high, and its function there so vital, that the brain takes up most of it.

DHA should not be confused with DHEA, which has been widely publicized in the media. DHEA is an acronym for *dehydroepiandrosterone*, the most abundant steroid hormone in the body. DHEA is the parent hormone for estrogen, testosterone, and cortisol. The biochemical and functional differences between DHA and DHEA are vast and complex.

Where DHA Is Most Concentrated in the Brain and Nervous System[9]

- Synaptosomes. Where nerve cells communicate with one another.
- Photoreceptors. The portion of the retina of the eye that receives light stimulation.
- Mitochondria. The generators of energy for all nerve cells.
- Cerebral cortex. The outer layer of the brain dense with cells rich in DHA

DHA is written in technical jargon as 22:6n3, meaning it has twenty-two carbons, six double bonds, and is an omega-3 fatty acid. These are the structural aspects that give DHA its unique place in the brain. It is a very long, electrically active fatty acid. The six double bonds give it a curved, spacious shape that provides for a fluid, supple nerve cell membrane. Other fatty acids come close, but none appear to share the unique properties of DHA. The spatial aspects of DHA appear to be important to hold the receptors in place within the nerve cell membranes. As described in Chapter Two, proper binding of neurotransmitters with receptors is essential for peak nerve communication.

When the brain does not receive enough DHA, it relies on a replacement fatty acid called DPA. According to Dr. C. D. Stubbs, "when cells are deprived of sources [of DHA] in the diet the cell will tend to produce the nearest fatty acid (in terms of unsaturation and chain length) that is possible, even if the fatty acid is from the omega-6 series."[10]

Replacing the brain's vital omega-3 fatty acid with an omega-6 fatty acid of different biochemical activity may be a great disadvantage, as we'll later see. If dietary fatty acid levels get too far out of balance, the brain often contains a peculiar omega-9 fatty acid called mead acid, which does not belong in the brain.[11]

As discussed previously, DHA is critical for the developing fetal brain and during infancy. Children who receive adequate DHA have been shown to have better visual acuity and IQ than children who receive inadequate amounts of this fatty acid.[12,13] These are periods when preformed DHA must be provided since the body during these periods in unable to make enough. As we age, actually as we pass age twenty, the enzymes that allow us to make our own DHA begin to wear out. In addition, DHA levels in the retina decrease with age.[14] We will explore evidence later in this book that low DHA in adulthood may even predispose one to early senility and poor cognitive function. These findings suggest that preformed DHA may be needed from the diet throughout life.

The most abundant sources of DHA include salmon, mackerel, herring, sardines, anchovies, and bluefin. Fish get their DHA by consuming microscopic marine algae. Therefore, some forms of algae are also good sources. In general, cold water fish contain more DHA than their warm water counterparts. There is some evidence that farmed fish such as salmon contain more DHA than wild fish.[15] This likely depends on the species and the dietary intake of the fish. Eggs contain variable amounts of DHA. However, if eggs are overcooked much of the DHA can be destroyed.

Mother's milk contains vastly more DHA than cow's milk, making mother's milk a far superior source of this nutrient for the infant and toddler brain.[16] Adults consuming cow's milk will receive large amounts of saturated fat, but no DHA needed by the brain. In Japan, DHA is considered so important to human health that it is now used to enrich more than twenty different foods.[17]

Who Gets Enough DHA?

There are many groups of people that do not get adequate DHA in their diets. Recent studies have shown that vegetarians are among these because they consume no animal foods and thus no preformed DHA in their diets. In a study of the blood levels of long-chain fatty acids of vegetarians, doctors found that DHA levels were very low, especially in long-term vegetarians.[18] When studying the effects of mothers' vegetarian diet on the fatty acid levels of newborns researchers found there to be less DHA in the blood of infants.[19] This would also suggest that the mother's DHA levels might be low. Another group of researchers found the DHA levels of breast-fed infants of vegetarian mothers to be only about one-third the level of breast-fed infants of mothers who consumed meat *and* vegetables.[20]

We might conclude from this that men, women, and children who are strict vegetarians may need to supplement their diets with DHA. This may be especially important for women of childbearing age, pregnant mothers, and nursing mothers. From the evidence above it may also be critical to get enhanced levels of DHA for many months after giving birth to a child. Plant-based DHA supplements are now available that should address the fatty acid needs of vegetarians without compromising their philosophical beliefs. (See Chapter Twelve.)

Many people who consume meat in their diets also get no DHA because their diets are devoid of cold water fish, a principal source of DHA. Their diets are also low in foods that contain the precursor to DHA, alpha-linolenic acid. Such individuals must also modify their diets to get adequate preformed DHA.

ALA: PARENT OF THE MAJOR BRAIN FAT DHA

As mentioned above, ALA, or alpha-linolenic acid, is an omega-3 fatty acid that must be present in order for the body to make its own DHA. Several studies have shown that ALA inadequacy can lead to poor DHA formation and poor brain and nerve function. Supplementation with ALA has been shown to increase DHA levels in the brain in some circumstances. ALA is important in the messenger functions of the body. It is converted into EPA (eicosapentaenoic acid) and then into PGE3 (prostaglandin E3). This important messenger, as we've seen, helps reduce platelet clumping and relaxes blood vessels. It is helpful in balancing immune function and inflammation. Without adequate ALA, we may be unable to properly regulate our PGE3 messengers. Thus, in the overall scheme, it is important to provide adequate ALA in the diet on a regular basis.

While consuming ALA provides the raw material needed to make our own DHA, we will see in Chapter Five that there are many things that can upset the process of making DHA. In fact, it has been estimated that perhaps 100 molecules of ALA are ingested for every molecule of DHA that is made. Also recall that those who consume too much of the omega-6 oils may be less efficient at making their own DHA. This may mean that, for some people, merely getting enough ALA is not adequate. They may need ALA *and* DHA to ensure adequate nutrition for their brains and nervous systems. We will see later that there are many studies and cases in which supplementation with ALA has helped people with certain brain-related conditions such as hyperactivity, aggression, depression, learning difficulties, neuropathy, and tinnitus.

While ALA itself is not found in the brain, it is widely distributed throughout other body cells. Therefore, adequate daily ALA is important to general health and well being.

Where ALA is Found in Food

Alpha-linolenic acid is found in a small number of foods. It is most abundant in flax seed oil and hemp seed oil. Walnut, pumpkin seed, and green leafy vegetables all contain varying amounts of ALA, though much less than flax and hemp. It used to be found in soybean oil, but hybridization has made most of the soybean oils deficient in ALA. Many of these sources of ALA were staple foods early in this century. Modern dietary practices have made this fatty acid scarce.

EPA: HELPING THE BRAIN'S BLOOD AND MESSENGERS

EPA, or eicosapentaenoic acid, is a long-chain fatty acid that is found throughout the body. EPA is not found in the brain in any appreciable amounts and is, therefore, not usually considered among the brain-fats. It has a significant effect on the messengers called eicosanoids. By virtue of these messengers, EPA influences inflammation, immune function, blood vessel activity, blood clotting, and the brain's blood supply.

EPA has been studied in a wide range of inflammatory conditions and has shown tremendous benefit. Since it is only found in trace amounts in the brain, its role there is not clear. Some infants who received fish oil experienced slight reductions in growth leading some doctors to wonder whether EPA displaced too much arachidonic acid from the body's cells. Adults taking EPA do not have the same general conerns since modern dietary practices commonly result in arachidonic acid levels already too high.

EPA is found in the same foods as DHA, though often in higher amounts than DHA. Many people wishing to increase DHA levels in their diet take fish oil capsules as a source. For many people this may be a reasonable practice and will produce great benefit. However, if one wishes to consume DHA solely with the intent to supply this important brain fatty acid, a supplemental source of only DHA may be desirable. For infants and small children, this may be especially important.

Whenever EPA intake is increased, antioxidants such as vitamin E must be consumed. This helps prevent damage to the delicate long-chain fatty acid molecules.

AA: THE JEKYLL AND HYDE OF BRAIN-FATS

AA, or arachidonic acid, is unique in that it is abundant in brain cells as well as in other body cells. Arachidonic acid is a long chain unsaturated fatty acid that is the principal fatty acid of the omega-6 family found in the brain. It consists of twenty carbons and four double bonds, so it is shorter and less unsaturated than DHA. In a developing fetus, AA is taken from the mother to help develop the fetal brain. In infancy, arachidonic acid is present in breast milk to further promote brain development. At about one year, a child is normally able to make enough of its own arachidonic acid. Thus, for the adult, *dietary* arachidonic acid is no longer as important.

Arachidonic acid levels in the brain are very carefully controlled. Arachidonic acid is found primarily in the fat of land animals such as beef, pork, chicken, and turkey, although shark oil, cod liver oil, squid, peanuts, and a few species of seaweed and algae have some. We can also make arachidonic acid from dietary linoleic acid.

This brings us to the Jekyll and Hyde aspect of arachidonic acid. Arachidonic acid is a precursor to many highly inflammatory substances, as discussed in Chapter Three. When arachidonic acid levels are too high in the lipids of cell membranes, there is a tendency toward formation of these inflammatory substances.

Reactive Substances Derived from Arachidonic Acid

Prostaglandin E2: Causes pain, swelling, inflammation.
Leukotriene: Causes pain, inflammation, movement of white blood cells to site of injury.
Thromboxane A2: Causes platelet stickiness (clotting) and blood vessel spasm.
Prostacyclin: Causes blood vessel relaxation and reduced platelet stickiness.

If we look at the typical American diet, it is rich with animal fat, high in omega-6 fatty acids, and low in omega-3 fatty acids. This is precisely the formula one would use if the wish was to promote inflammation and alter brain chemistry in a negative way.

Omega-3 fatty acids like EPA or DHA help to prevent excess arachidonic acid from accumulating in tissues. Sometimes, they are given therapeutically for the purpose of reducing arachidonic acid in the body. In this way, they help control or regulate inflammation and tissue damage. However, it is important to know that maintaining the levels of AA in the brain is also vital to brain function. Our goal should be to keep the level of arachidonic acid in balance with other fatty acids. This means we should consume foods that are low in arachidonic acid and low in linoleic acid, while balancing our omega-3 fatty acid intake.

GLA: MODIFYING THE BRAIN MESSENGERS

GLA, or gamma-linolenic acid, is not a true brain-fat because it is not used in forming the brain's structure—it is not part of the nerve cell membrane. The reason GLA appears to help in neuro-logical conditions is because it is converted into a substance known as PGE1, a hormonelike substance that has a powerful effect on some of the brain's functions. Encouraging the production of PGE1 can reduce the production of inflammatory substances that come from arachidonic acid.

GLA has been studied in a number of behavioral and neuro-logical conditions. For example, there are about 3,000 patients with multiple sclerosis (MS) currently taking evening primrose oil (a source of GLA) with good results. Dr. Richard Passwater has commented that fifteen to twenty percent of MS patients may receive significant benefit from GLA, while another 20 percent may receive some benefit.[21] GLA is only one factor in MS, so it is logi-cal that this oil alone would not improve symptoms in all MS suf-ferers.

Alcoholics may suffer from depression and mood swings, in part, because their bodies do not make enough of the hormone PGE1. When GLA is given, PGE1 formation is often enhanced and mood improves. Some children with hyperactivity or atten-tion deficit benefit enormously from GLA.[22] Schizophrenics may benefit from GLA supplementation. Also, some women who suf-fer from mood swings associated with premenstrual syndrome achieve significant improvement in mood with GLA.[23]

Gamma-linolenic acid is commonly used when we suspect an individual's enzymes are not properly converting their essential fatty acids to the messengers. Giving GLA allows us to "leapfrog" over the enzyme and provide the next fatty acid in the pathway. Once the body has GLA, it can often continue the conversion process of making the body's messenger PGE1. This is important in many conditions of illness as well as in infancy.

Gamma-linolenic acid is an omega-6 fatty acid (don't confuse it with *alpha*-linolenic acid, which is an omega-3 fatty acid). Com-mon sources include oil of borage seed, evening primrose, and black current seed.

MAKING THE CONVERSION

In order for the body to make fatty acids like DHA from dietary essential fatty acids like ALA, it must have enzymes. (Figure 9) The enzymes used in this process are called delta-5-desaturase and delta-6-desaturase.

These enzymes remain dormant until they are called to action. The call to action merely requires that the raw material, the fatty acid, be present. However, in order to actually do their work they need a series of cofactors to start the engine. These cofactors are usually in the form of vitamins and minerals. Without the cofactors, the enzymes don't become activated and the essential fatty acids are not converted properly into their long-chain neural fatty acids.

In this way, you might have the fatty acids you need, but you can't activate the enzymes because another nutrient is missing. We will explore these nutrients and other factors that affect the enzymes in the next chapter.

CHOLESTEROL IS NOT A DIRTY WORD: YOUR BRAIN NEEDS IT

Ever since cholesterol was associated with heart disease, it has developed an undeservedly negative reputation. Doctors advocated that patients refrain from eating eggs and avoid high cholesterol foods at every turn. The marketing of commercial foods touts the fact that this or that product "contains no cholesterol" or is "low in cholesterol." There is no doubt that when cholesterol in blood is too high it can lead to problems. But have we taken this notion too far?

In order to make the myelin sheath that covers your nerves, cholesterol is an absolutely essential molecule. In fact, cholesterol comprises an amazing one-fourth of the total lipids found in myelin. In order for membranes of the brain to remain stable, cholesterol is required. Vary the cholesterol too high or too low and you vary the fluidity of nerve membranes. Vary the fluidity and you change the properties of the membrane. In short, cholesterol is neither good, nor bad. Cholesterol is cholesterol. Imbalance in

Figure 9
How the Brain's Fatty Acids Are Made

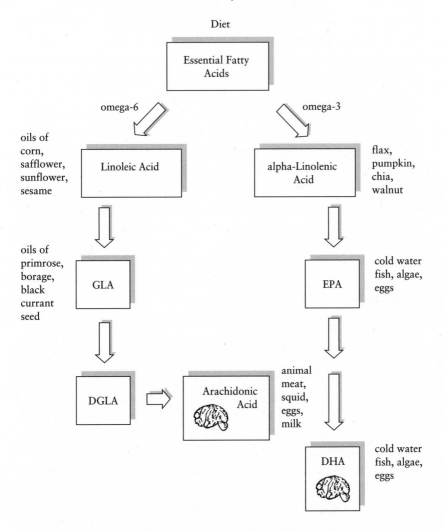

Diet

Essential Fatty
Acids

omega-6

omega-3

oils of
corn,
safflower,
sunflower,
sesame

Linoleic Acid

alpha-Linolenic
Acid

flax,
pumpkin,
chia,
walnut

oils of
primrose,
borage,
black
currant
seed

GLA

EPA

cold water
fish, algae,
eggs

DGLA

Arachidonic
Acid

animal
meat,
squid,
eggs,
milk

DHA

cold water
fish, algae,
eggs

either direction, high or low, leads to possible dysfunction and disease.

Cholesterol is also the raw material for making the vital steroid hormones DHEA, estrogen, progesterone, testosterone, and cortisol. Estrogen is a so-called female hormone, while testosterone is a so-called male hormone that triggers development of body hair, aggressiveness, superior muscle strength, and other traits. In reality, both hormones are present in both men and women. From the very beginning of life testosterone and estrogen influence the development and function of the brain. As we grow up and as we age, testosterone and estrogen levels even seem to influence mental function.[24]

Beyond the concerns about estrogen and testosterone, are there other obvious brain-related problems associated with low cholesterol? Do people even exist whose cholesterol is too low? The answer to both questions is "yes." In one study, male psychiatric patients with cholesterol in the lowest one fourth of the group were more than twice as likely to have made a serious suicide attempt than those with higher cholesterol.[25] We should also remember that myelin is seventy-five percent fat and that one-fourth of this must be cholesterol. For now, recognize that, for most people, cholesterol must not be avoided. It must be consumed rationally and in balance. This is especially true for the brain.

The Much-Maligned Egg

This brings us to the nagging question of the egg-cholesterol controversy. Should we continue to follow the admonition to avoid eggs because of their high cholesterol content? Two recent studies have strongly challenged this notion. In one study, up to three eggs per day were consumed for eight weeks with no significant rise in cholesterol. In another, up to four eggs were consumed each day for eight weeks with no significant rise in cholesterol. The researchers did not advocate a high egg diet, but stated that "some healthy individuals can pay less attention to their egg consumption if they maintain a low cholesterol level and low heart disease risk profile."[26]

Incidentally, the body puts such a high priority on cholesterol that it manufactures roughly 3,000 milligrams per day, about the amount contained in one dozen eggs. Moreover, eggs are one of the rare land-animal sources of DHA and an excellent source of lecithin (phosphatidylcholine).

ANOTHER FAMILY OF BRAIN-FATS: THE PHOSPHOLIPIDS

In Chapter Two, I discussed the role of essential fatty acids in formation of the nerve cell membrane. Key substances that form the bricks and mortar of these membranes are substances about which you will continue to hear a great deal. These are the phospholipids. *Phospho* means they contain the mineral phosphorous. *Lipid* means they contain fat molecules. Thus, phospholipid simply means substances that have both fat and phosphorous.

In the phospholipid, there are usually two fatty acid molecules: one saturated and one unsaturated. In the phospholipids of the brain, the unsaturated fatty acid is usually DHA or AA. Phospholipids are important in forming nerve membranes and in protecting nerve membranes from toxic injury and free radical attack.[27,28,29] Two common phospholipids are called phosphatidylcholine (PC, or lecithin) and phosphatidylserine (PS).

Phospholipids found in nutritional supplements are structurally similar to the phospholipids of nerve membranes. Because of this, supplemental phospholipids are increasingly being used as treatments in such things as memory-enhancement, depression, attention deficit disorder, schizophrenia, Alzheimer's disease, and Down syndrome. According to Harvard physician Dr. Margarita Woodbury, "In approximately 347 patients with neuropsychiatric disorders treated with choline or lecithin, 106 showed significant improvement, 61 demonstrated partial improvement, and 80 showed no changes. Thus, almost half exhibit some response."[30] There are now over thirty-four human studies on phosphatidylserine as applied to problems of memory and other brain-related conditions.[31]

TESTING FOR FATTY ACID IMBALANCE

Signs and symptoms can be helpful road maps that may suggest whether fats and oils are out of balance. While useful, they don't tell us much about which fatty acids are out of balance. To more precisely determine the levels of specific fatty acids in an individual requires a blood test. In this test, red blood cells are analyzed for their fatty acid content. The laboratory reports on the major saturated and unsaturated fatty acids, the ratios between omega-6 and omega-3 fatty acids, and relative percentages of each unsaturated fatty acid.

It is important that red blood cells be used rather than serum or plasma because the information gives a better reflection of what is happening in the body. One drawback of using blood to test for fatty acid status is that it does not give a measure of *brain* fatty acids. However, since getting a sample of brain tissue is out of the question, measuring red cell fatty acids is the best we currently have. Despite this limitation, red cell fatty acid analysis is *extremely* valuable in deciphering the unique fatty acid needs of an individual. (Appendix B contains a list of laboratories that perform fatty acid analysis.)

For example, Lucas struggled with moodiness, aggressive outbursts, inattentiveness, and difficulty concentrating. Fatty acid analysis of his red blood cells showed the following:

ALA	Low
EPA	Low
DHA	Low
GLA	Low
Stearic (saturated)	High
Elaidic (trans)	High
AA to EPA ratio	High
Polyunsaturated to Saturated ratio	Low

From this profile, we can quickly see that all of his omega-3 fatty acids were too low, his saturated fats too high, and trans fatty acids too high. His ratio of arachidonic acid to EPA was too high, which does not bode particularly well for the inflammatory system or brain messenger system. His ratio of polyunsaturated fatty acids to saturated fatty acids is too low.

This profile was extremely valuable because it showed us what was happening in his body and allowed us to design a program tailored specifically to his needs. Lucas needed to drastically reduce his intake of saturated fats and trans fatty acids. He needed to increase all of the omega-3 fatty acids, especially DHA. He also needed to address factors that help his enzymes convert dietary fatty acids into their active substances and longer chain fatty acids required by the brain.

In addition to red cell fatty acid analysis, it is now possible to test a mother's breast milk to see if it contains adequate fatty acids to nourish her nursing child's brain. From the lab test one can develop a supplementation plan that is very specific to the needs of mother and child.

SIGNS OF FATTY ACID IMBALANCE

Fatty acid imbalance can manifest in many different ways and may affect almost any body system. However, there is set of signs and symptoms that many doctors agree to be correlated with fatty acid imbalance. We should pay particularly close attention to the skin signs and symptoms.

Dry skin	Dry, unmanageable hair
Dandruff	Excessive thirst
Frequent urination	Brittle, easily frayed nails
Irritability	Hyperactivity
Attention deficit	"Chicken skin" on backs of arms
Soft nails	Dry eyes
Alligator skin	Learning problems
Allergies	Poor wound healing
Lowered immunity	Frequent infections
Weakness	Patches of pale skin on cheeks
Fatigue	Cracked skin on heels or fingertips

In the next chapter, we will explore some of the companion nutrients needed to make the fatty acid system work properly. We will also see the boulders in the path to peak fatty acid balance.

CHAPTER 5

MAKING THE SYSTEM WORK

Consuming the right balance of fats and oils significantly improves the odds for better brain health. However, the vagaries of modern life raise the chance that boulders may lie in the path. There are four important factors that determine how well our fatty acid system works. They are:

- Healthy digestion and absorption
- Key nutrients that make the enzymes of fatty acid conversion work
- Dietary and lifestyle factors that block the enzymes
- Sugars and carbohydrates that rev up the arachidonic acid inflammatory system

THE IMPORTANCE OF HEALTHY DIGESTION

In order to make use of the fatty acids you get from your diet, your food must first be digested and absorbed. Digestion is the process by which enzymes in your digestive tract break down foods into smaller and smaller components. Absorption is the process by which your body transfers the nutrients from the intestinal tract into the bloodstream. If either one of these processes isn't working properly you may not get the fatty acids you need.

The importance of this was illustrated by doctors at Boston University School of Medicine. They recently showed that people with digestive problems resulting in malabsorption or diarrhea were much more likely to have essential fatty acid deficiency and essential fatty acid insufficiency. People with a condition called Crohn's disease had the poorest fatty acid status.[1] Clinical experience has shown that there are many other circumstances in which digestion and absorption are impaired enough to alter fatty acid status.

Darryl had suffered from symptoms of tremors and muscle weakness for about five years. It was evident from blood profiles that he had essential fatty acid imbalance. However, when he took fatty acids he experienced soft stools and digestive discomfort. Follow-up testing of digestive function revealed that he had low pancreatic enzymes and excessive fat in his stools. In essence, he was not breaking fat down into its smaller components nor was he efficiently absorbing the fat into his bloodstream. He had a further problem of bacterial overgrowth in the small intestine. His path to recovery consisted of taking digestive enzymes to improve the breakdown of fat and a plant-based antibacterial to eradicate the harmful intestinal bacteria. He also took acidophilus and bifidus to restore normal populations of helpful bacteria to his bowel. With this program he was able not only to tolerate the fatty acids, but showed significant improvement in his neurological symptoms.

This case is reminiscent of young Derek who suffered from hyperactivity and attention problems. He had a long history of antibiotic use, which seemed to contribute to the abdominal cramping, bloating, and gas he experienced. Stool analysis revealed a parasite known as cryptosporidium. Derek also had classic signs of fatty acid imbalance: frequent urination, increased thirst, and dry skin. Blood tests (IgG) for food allergies revealed a number of items to which he was allergic. His treatment required attention to parasitic infection, bacterial imbalance, food allergies, poor digestion, and essential fatty acids. Recovery on this program was slow, but his progress was steady and led to a much-improved quality of life.

Both cases serve as gentle reminders that some problems are no so simple as a fatty acid supplement. It is not at all uncommon to have to attend to digestive function before noticing improvement in someone's condition.

In addition to fatty acids, vitamin E is another important nutrient in brain function. Vitamin E, being a fat-soluble nutrient, is sometimes poorly absorbed when problems exist with the gallbladder, pancreas, small intestine, or other components of the digestive tract. In disorders of the gastrointestinal tract, vitamin E deficiency may develop and lead to a number of brain and nervous system signs and symptoms such as abnormal reflexes, loss of pain and touch sensation, muscle weakness, movement and balance problems, and visual disturbance.[2]

Factors That May Impair Digestion and Absorption

Some of those listed alter digestion while others impair absorption:

Antacids	Inadequate chewing
Antibiotics	Bacteria
Viruses	Protozoan (parasites)
Fungi	Yeast
Food intolerance	Poor nutrition (esp. fatty acids)
Alcohol	Anti-inflammatory drugs (aspirin, indomethacin)

Food intolerance can significantly affect digestion and absorption. Whenever digestive problems exist, food allergy or intolerance should be considered. The most common offending foods are dairy products, wheat, soy, peanuts, eggs, and corn. However, many other foods can cause difficulty in an individual. Food allergies may also trigger the release of inflammatory messengers made from arachidonic acid. In this way, food allergies may modify inflammatory pathways and even affect brain function. Identification and removal of offending foods from the diet can be an important part of the recovery process in some people.

Fatty Acids and Digestion

One needs a healthy digestive system in order to absorb dietary fats and oils. Paradoxically, however, the integrity of the cells lining the digestive tract depends upon fatty acids. In Chapter Two, I discussed the importance of essential fatty acids in forming cell membranes throughout the body. The small intestine, where most nutrient absorption takes place, is lined with billions of cells, each of which has a membrane made of essential fatty acids. The surface area of the small intestine is roughly the size of a tennis court, so one can imagine that a large amount of essential fatty acids are needed to maintain its structure.

Every few days, the cells lining the small intestine slough off and are replaced by new cells. Every time a new cell replaces an old cell, essential fatty acids are required to build the new cell membrane. The fats that go into your mouth are the very same fats that will be used to form the new cell membranes.

If the diet does not contain adequate essential fatty acids, the intestinal membranes will not contain adequate EFAs and rebuilding will be difficult. As a result, absorption of nutrients can be a problem. Repairing the intestinal cells requires linoleic acid, GLA, ALA, and EPA. There is very little DHA used in the intestinal lining and there is often too much arachidonic acid in an inflamed intestinal tract.

Not only do fatty acids form the *structure* of the intestinal cells, they also form messengers such as those described in Chapter Three. If intestinal cells contain too much omega-6 and too little of the omega-3 fatty acids, they may be primed for inflammation.[3] Balancing fats and oils can help maintain the integrity of the membranes of the digestive tract and maintain healthy absorption.

MAKING THE BRAIN-FATS AND MESSENGERS: VITAMIN AND MINERAL NEEDS

Several vitamins and minerals are important in the path that essential fatty acids take to become either messengers (prostaglandins, eicosanoids, etc.) or brain-fats (DHA, AA) (Figure 10). Failure to get enough of these nutrients may mean that the body's ability to regulate its formation of the right fatty acids and messengers, according to its needs, may be impaired. The main nutrients needed for this conversion include:

Recommended Dietary Allowance (RDA) of Selected Nutrients

Nutrient	Age 0–3	4–6	7–18	Adult	Pregnant	Lactating
Vitamin B6	0.3–1.0 mg	1.1 mg	1.4–2.0 mg	1.6 mg	2.1 mg	1.6 mg
Vitamin B3	5–9 mg	12 mg	13–20 mg	15 mg	20 mg	15 mg
Vitamin C	30–40 mg	45 mg	60 mg	60 mg	95 mg	60 mg
Magnesium	40–80 mg	120 mg	120 mg	280 mg	355 mg	280 mg
Zinc	5–10 mg	10 mg	10–15 mg	12 mg	19 mg	12 mg

Note that these values are only estimated values thought to be the minimum required to prevent deficiency disease. There is considerable debate as to whether these levels are adequate to promote *optimum health*. In fact, many nutrition scientists believe that the levels needed for optimum health are far above those listed in the RDA. (See suggested levels below.) Even if we use the RDA as a standard, it is clear that many Americans do not get enough of these critical nutrients.

For example, in a survey of Americans, only twenty-five percent had a dietary intake of magnesium that equaled or exceeded the RDA.[4] The dietary intake of magnesium for pregnant women in the U.S. is only thirty-five to fifty-eight percent of the recommended dietary allowance.[5] Of those with chemical sensitivity, forty percent were magnesium deficient.[6] In one study of American men and women, sixty-eight percent were found to consume less than two thirds of the RDA for zinc.[7] In a government study of adults aged nineteen to seventy-four, ninety percent of women and seventy-one percent of men consumed less than the RDA for vitamin B6.[8] B6 was found to be marginally deficient in fifty percent of pregnant women and it was estimated that a supplement of 20 mg per day may be needed to keep the blood levels of B6 normal.[9]

Ensuring peak function of the fatty acid pathways may require far higher levels of nutrients than described in the RDA.

Suggested Optimal Nutrient Levels for Brain-Fat Formation

Nutrient	Children	Adults	Pregnancy	Lactating
Vitamin B6	2–10mg	10–25mg	10–100 mg*	10–100mg*
Vitamin B3	15–40mg	30–50mg	30–50mg	30–50mg
Vitamin C	500–1,000mg	500–2,000mg	500–2,000mg	500–2,000mg
Magnesium	100–200mg	400–800mg	400–800mg	400–800mg
Zinc	10–20mg	15–30mg	15–30mg	15–30mg

* More than 150–200mg of B6 may suppress lactation.

Vitamin B12 is critical for brain function and should also be considered when fatty acid problems exist or brain-related problems exist. Other nutrients such as potassium, chloride, and selenium may be important as well. However, supplementation with these is much trickier and should be based on laboratory tests.

THE BRAIN FAT BLOCKERS:
FACTORS THAT PREVENT YOU FROM MAKING YOUR OWN BRAIN-FATS

While your body needs cofactor nutrients to run the enzymes that help you make your own brain-fat DHA, there are a number of things that may block this process. Understanding these can help you construct a diet and lifestyle that help you maximize your ability to make your own brain-fats.

Factors that Block the Delta-6-desaturase Enzymes[10]

- High dietary or blood cholesterol
- High dietary saturated fat
- High trans fatty acid intake (See Chapter Seven)
- Stress
- Alcohol consumption
- Diabetes
- Atopy (an inherited predisposition to allergies, eczema, etc.)
- Sugar (See below)
- Infancy (Enzyme is not active until about age one. This is one reason infants need preformed fats like GLA and DHA.)

Figure 10
Making the Enzymes of Fatty Acid Conversion Work

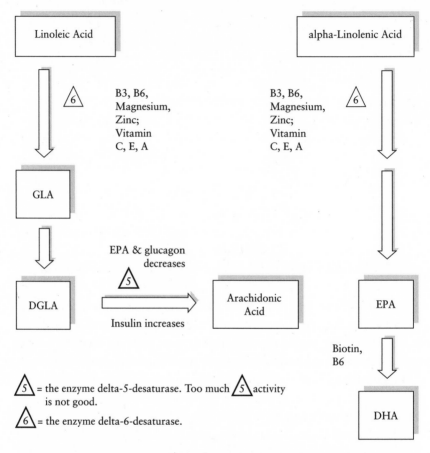

$\triangle 5$ = the enzyme delta-5-desaturase. Too much $\triangle 5$ activity is not good.

$\triangle 6$ = the enzyme delta-6-desaturase.

Dietary fatty acids are converted by enzymes into their long-chain products that are ultimately used in forming the brain's structure. The enzymes can be assisted or blocked by many factors.

- Aging (After the twenties the enzymes slowly decline in efficiency.)
- Medication such as corticosteroids and non-steroidal anti-inflammatory drugs (aspirin, indomethacin, ibuprofen, etc.)
- Various genetic errors where the enzyme is not fully active
- Elevated blood glucose or insulin
- Obesity

- Smoking
- Fasting or starvation

EASY ON THE ALCOHOL

Alcohol poses significant problems to the brain's fatty acid pathways. It blocks the enzymes needed to form DHA and also blocks the enzyme needed to form PGE1. Further, alcohol appears to dissolve fatty acids within the brain's membranes. This, in fact, may be one of the reasons for the mental impairment that gradually sets in with alcohol consumption.

Dr. R. J. Pawlosky, of the National Intitutes of Health, has studied the affect of alcohol on the nervous system and notes that alcohol causes a decrease in DHA in the brain's membranes. The DHA is replaced by a poor substitute known as DPA. He acknowledges that this change may bode ill for the brain since "Studies of lower concentrations of DHA (22:6n3) in the nervous system is associated with a loss of nervous system function."[11] Dr. Norman Salem has suggested that alcoholics, as part of their recovery, may require DHA supplementation in order to restore the brain fatty acids that have been damaged over the years.[12]

Pawlosky writes, "Alcoholics are prone to many cognitive disorders involving loss of memory, inability to concentrate, and dementia. Some of these functions may be modulated, in part, by DHA concentrations. The alcohol-induced loss of neural DHA may provide a mechanism underlying aspects of this neurological impairment." Pawolsky's comments refer to alcoholics, but there is reason to think that more moderate consumption of alcohol may also come with a price of some form.

The damage to neural fatty acids may also explain some of the brain damage that occurs to fetuses whose mothers consume alcohol during pregnancy. Mothers who are pregnant should absolutely refrain from alcohol.

WATCH YOUR SUGARS:
CONCERNS ABOUT HIGH CARBOHYDRATE DIETS

Another factor that may disrupt your ability to properly use and make the fatty acids needed by your brain is too much sugar, too much complex carbohydrate, or the wrong kind of complex carbohydrate.

When you consume sugars your body secretes more insulin. Insulin is a hormone that helps move your sugar out of the blood and into your body cells. Insulin also, however, affects the enzymes that convert essential fatty acids. If you have too much insulin your enzymes that convert gamma-linolenic acid (GLA) to arachidonic acid may become more active. If you make too much arachidonic acid your body is primed for inflammation. In addition, your brain may produce too much PGE2, which can affect a range of functions. For this reason, it is important that you control your sugar and starch intake. This includes simple sugars and also certain kinds of complex sugars.

Different carbohydrates affect your blood sugar differently. The measure of this effect is called the glycemic index. The higher the glycemic index of a food the more stress it places on your blood sugar control, your insulin response, and your fatty acid control. Lower glycemic index foods place less of this stress on these systems and promote better health overall.

Below is a list of the glycemic index of many common foods. You should try to eat foods with a low glycemic index and minimize or eliminate the high glycemic index foods. Whenever you consume such foods, they can be consumed with a fatty meal to slow delivery to the bloodstream.

Try to ensure that carbohydrates comprise no more than forty percent of your diet and that those used on a regular basis have a glycemic index below fifty. Higher glycemic index foods may result in a lower blood sugar response when consumed with adequate fat, which slows their delivery to the blood stream. Commonly, more highly processed carbohydrates have a higher glycemic index.

Approximate Glycemic Index of Selected Foods[13,14]

Sugars

Glucose	138
Fructose	26
Sucrose	83

Breakfast Cereals

All-bran	74
Cornflakes	121
Muesli	96
Oatmeal	89
Shredded Wheat	97

Dried Legumes

Beans (canned)	60
Beans (kidney)	43
Beans (soy)	20
Peas (black-eyed)	45
Chickpeas	46
Lentils	36

Fruit

Apples	50-60
Bananas	84
Oranges	59
Orange juice	71
Raisins	93

Grains and Cereal Products

Buckwheat	68
Bread (white)	100
Bread (whole grain)	100
Millet	103
Rice (brown)	81
Rice (white)	54
Spaghetti (whole grain)	61
Spaghetti (white)	67
Sweet corn	80

Vegetables

Frozen peas	51
Beets	64
Carrots	92
Parsnips	97
Potato (new)	80
Potato (sweet)	70
Yam	74

Dairy Products

Ice cream	69
Milk (non-fat)	46
Milk (whole)	44
Yogurt	52

GETTING THE PROTEIN YOU NEED, WITHOUT THE FAT

Getting adequate protein is an important part of a healthy diet. However, many sources of protein contain high amounts of fat. The fat that accompanies many animal proteins is often arachidonic acid, which you do not want in excess. To keep the arachidonic acid levels in your diet in check, generally consume lean meat products that are low in fat. Ideally, these would also be organic meats. Fish is the best animal protein because, in addition to providing protein, some species* also provide omega-3 fatty acids. Animal protein sources that might be considered include:

Fish

Salmon*, Mackerel,* Herring*, Sardines* Tuna*, Bass, Cod, Trout*, Swordfish, Haddock.

Fowl

Turkey breast, skinless (organic, range fed preferable); chicken breast, skinless (organic, range fed preferable), duck, partridge, pheasant, and other wild game. Chickens raised on an algae-based chicken feed called *DHA Gold* have five to seven times the DHA of normal chickens. This should be noted on the label in stores.

Beef and Pork

Limit beef and pork products. If you use these, make sure they are lean, less than 10 percent fat. Poor choices in this category are sausages, fatty cuts of beef or pork (more than 15 percent fat), bacon, hot dogs, and salami.

Eggs

Organic eggs from free-range chickens contain protein, DHA, phosphatidylcholine, and other rich nutrients beneficial to the brain. Eggs from chickens raised on an algae-based chicken feed called *DHA Gold* contain much more DHA than eggs from normal chickens. This should be noted on the label in stores. Concerns about eggs and cholesterol, as noted in Chapter Four, are overstated for most healthy people. Remember, one-fourth of the lipid in brain cell myelin is cholesterol.

Dairy Products

Good choices, provided there is no allergy to dairy products, include low-fat cheese, low-fat and yogurt. These are cases where low-fat products are useful. Whole milk, ice-cream, and other milk products contain high amounts of saturated fat. In addition, they contain arachidonic acid. They are acceptable for occasional use, but as a staple they provide neither the right kind nor the right balance of fats. For children, in whom the brain is still forming, regular consumption of dairy products fill them with protein and fat, but the fat is not conducive to peak brain formation.

HELPING THE PATHWAYS WORK THEIR BEST

To make sure that the path from the food on your plate to your brain is given the best chance at peak function, consider the following:

- Eat the right balance of fats and oils
- Make sure digestion and absorption are working well.
- Avoid the food, environmental, and lifestyle factors that block the fatty acid-converting enzymes.
- Make sure you get adequate amounts of the co-factors zinc, magnesium, vitamin B6, vitamin B3, and vitamin C. Also consider vitamins B12, folic acid, and biotin.
- Limit your intake of high sugar foods and those with a high glycemic index.
- Balance protein, fat, and carbohydrate. A general *starting point* might be the following, then tailor to your needs.
  - 40 percent of calories from carbohydrate
  - 30 percent of calories from protein
  - 30 percent of calories from fat assuming proper n-6/n-3 fatty acid balance

CHAPTER 6

IF THE BRAIN IS MOSTLY FAT, CAN IT GO RANCID?

That the brain is mostly fat is a fascinating prospect by itself. But this fact also raises one very provocative and intriguing question. Can the brain go rancid? Though at first glance the question may seem odd, if not ridiculous, closer inspection causes us to take it more seriously. In fact, the question of whether the brain can go rancid is one with which medical science has grappled for some time.

Virtually anything that contains unsaturated oils can become rancid. But what does rancid really mean? If you sent your rancid cooking oil to a laboratory, they would look for the footprints of damaged fatty acids. The term lipid peroxide is used to describe what happens in any polyunsaturated oil when oxygen has entered the fatty acid molecule in some way (you can think of lipid peroxides as oxygen-damaged fatty acids). When a fatty acid becomes a lipid peroxide (becomes rancid) the shape, structure, function, and activity of the fatty acid is profoundly changed.

To answer the question of whether the brain can go rancid we have to look at the ingredients needed for any oil to go rancid. They are:

1. Polyunsaturated oil.
2. Oxygen (air), heat, light, or other sources of free radicals.
3. Need for antioxidants to protect the fatty acid molecules.

1. The brain is rich in polyunsaturated fatty acids. In fact, the brain contains the highest concentration of DHA anywhere in the body. Recall that DHA is the longest and most unsaturated fatty acid known to play an important role in the body. The more unsaturated the fatty acid, the greater its susceptibility to becoming rancid. The order of susceptibility to rancidity, moving from highest to lowest, is:

Polyunsaturated >> Monounsaturated >> Saturated >> Cholesterol

Because the brain is so rich in long-chain polyunsaturated fatty acids it satisfies the first condition for susceptibility to rancidity.

2. Oxygen or other sources of free radicals. Oxygen is one of the most devastating molecules for unsaturated oils. Paradoxically, the brain is the most oxygen-hungry tissue in the body. Remember, the brain is only about six percent of your adult body weight, but uses about twenty percent of the body's oxygen to generate its energy. Reliance of such a delicate fatty structure on oxygen makes it very susceptible to damage. In addition to oxygen, there are many other sources of free radical stress that may affect the brain and nervous system.

Sources of Free Radicals That May Affect the Brain

Alcohol	Some drugs
Bacterial waste	Viruses
Smoking	Toxic metals (lead, mercury, cadmium)
Stress	Normal minerals in excess (iron, manganese, copper, etc.)
Food allergens	Toxic chemicals (benzene, toluene, etc.)
Diabetes	Liver disease
White blood cell activity	Intestinal dysbiosis (imbalance of gut organisms)
Certain amino acids (MSG)	Nutrient insufficiency
Trauma or injury	Normal oxygen-using activity

The brain easily satisfies the second condition because it is susceptible to free radicals and exposed to regular doses of oxygen and other free radical substances.

3. Need for protective antioxidants. Unsaturated oils in nature (plants and animals) are protected from going rancid by the existence of antioxidants. Oils in which the antioxidant content is low go rancid more quickly.

The brain relies on a complex network of antioxidants to protect its delicate fatty acids. In the brain, when the antioxidant balance is poor the brain fatty acids go rancid more quickly as well. While the brain is rich in some antioxidants like vitamins C and E, it is low in certain enzymatic antioxidants that would normally protect tissues from damage. These enzymes include catalase, glutathione peroxidase, and superoxide dismutase.[1] Therefore, the brain satisfies the third condition. It has a great need for and dependence upon antioxidants for its very survival.

In their book, *Free Radicals in Biology and Medicine,* Drs. Barry Halliwell and John Gutteridge devote over eighty pages to the subject of lipid peroxidation. Regarding the brain, they write, "The brain and nervous system may be especially prone to oxidant damage for a number of reasons."[2]

Another clue to the brain's susceptibility to rancidity lies in its energy system.

THE ENGINES OF BRAIN ENERGY

Living within each of our brain cells (and other cells) are tiny organelles called mitochondria. These microscopic entities exist to produce energy in the form of ATP (adenosine triphosphate). ATP is like the energy currency. It is the substance that allows all of the activities in your brain to take place. Without ATP your neurons would not conduct signals, your neurotransmitters would not be made, your brain would cease to function. The body is constantly making and breaking down ATP. In fact, ATP is so much a part of us that the total amount required for a day's work would weigh an estimated 150 to 200 pounds.

Because of this, some have argued that the most important enzyme in the body is a protein called sodium-potassium-activated ATPase (Na/K ATPase); we'll call it simply "ATPase." This enzyme controls the transfer of ions (sodium and potassium) during nerve transmission. In doing so, it consumes an astounding *one-half* of the entire energy used by the brain, or nearly a tenth of the energy of the whole body. Obviously, if this enzyme is not functioning at its best or is not present in adequate amounts, brain function suffers.

The cell membranes of mitochondria are rich in essential fatty acids. Once again, proper balance of fatty acids seems important. Experiments have shown that when the intake of alpha-linolenic acid (the precursor to DHA) is restricted, the level of ATPase in the nerve endings falls by one-half. Some studies have shown that such deficiencies are clearly enough to slow nerve conduction in the brain and in peripheral nerves. After only four weeks of restricting alpha-linolenic acid from the diet, there are dramatic changes in the retina. In fact, it takes as much as ten times more light to get the eyes to respond.[3]

The Stray Sparks of Brain Energy

The intense energy-producing activity taking place within the brain sometimes comes with a price. When mitochondria conduct their energy-producing affairs, there is always some electron leakage. You might liken these to sparks from a fire. The body seems to tolerate low-level electron leakage. However, under certain circumstances, excessive electrons may leak out of mitochondria. If not properly contained, such leakage can lead to damage of surrounding tissues or poisoning of the mitochondria themselves.

It is a somewhat like burning a fire in a fireplace. Logs are burned to generate energy in the form of heat, but occasional embers may leap from the fire. The fire screen normally protects the home from leaping embers. However, should the fire screen be left ajar, leaping embers may actually set the curtains ablaze and threaten the entire house.

In nerve cell mitochondria, it is the antioxidant nutrients and enzymes that keep the stray electrons from damaging the delicate unsaturated fatty acids of the cell membranes. Yet, if the mitochondria are not working efficiently, they may "leak" more free radicals into their surroundings than is normal and further tax the antioxidant system. Stray electrons from mitochondria may damage their own DNA, their energy-making ability, and thus, the brain cells themselves. This is one factor that may cause rancid fats within the brain.

When Stray Sparks Damage the Nerves

Researchers are now beginning to discover that damage to the mitochondria occuring in brain tissue might be responsible for the damage that occurs in some brain disorders. In one study, Alzheimer's patients had much higher damage to their mitochondrial DNA than people without Alzheimer's.[4] Dr. Flint Beal, at Massachusetts General Hospital in Boston, has suggested that defects in brain neuron mitochondria might predispose people to neurodegenerative disease later in life.[5] Dr. W. Davis Parker of the University of Virginia School of Medicine, has stated, "I think the evidence that mitochondria play a role in neurodegenerative disease is stronger than ever."[6]

We do not entirely understand how to protect nerve cells from damage, but we do know of some preventive steps that can help. We must keep the energy machinery working efficiently. This can be done with specific nutrition to some extent. Next, we must make sure that antioxidant levels are adequate.

NUTRIENTS THAT SUPPORT BRAIN ENERGY PRODUCTION

Various nutrients have been shown to help make the production of energy more efficient within the brain's mitochondria. This may help keep the brain's neurons functioning more efficiently and prevent the damaging effects of stray electrons. Providing these nutrients in supplemental doses may eventually prove to be supportive for people with nervous system conditions. For the average healthy person who wants to seek optimal health and peak brain power, ensuring a diet adequate in these nutrients may be important. The nutrients listed below (except anthocyanadins) have known roles in mitochondria.

Nutrients That Support Brain Energy [7,8,9,10,11,12,13]

Coenzyme Q10	N- acetyl carnitine
N-acetyl cysteine	Lipoic acid
Glutathione	Vitamin C
Thiamin	Vitamin E (mixed tocopherols)
Riboflavin	Anthocyanadins
Magnesium	Essential fatty acids

DEFENDING THE BRAIN'S FATS: THE ANTIOXIDANT SYSTEM

Recognizing the unique susceptibility of the brain's fats to go rancid makes our discussion of antioxidants more compelling. Scientists have shown, for example, that the level of lipid peroxides in senile dementia is elevated. Even the aging process appears to increase the level of lipid peroxides in the brain.[14]

Several studies have explored the capacity of antioxidants to protect the nervous system. Parkinson's disease is a condition where a portion of the brain that controls movement is slowly destroyed. There is no single cause of Parkinson's disease and numerous factors appear capable of damaging a tiny area called the substantia nigra. Even though there is no single cause, doctors have begun to observe a pattern of free-radical damage.

At the Columbia University Department of Neurology, physicians gave high doses of vitamin E and vitamin C daily to Parkinson's patients. The strategy was based on evidence that free radicals might be at work and that antioxidant nutrients might slow the damage from free radicals. The individuals receiving this therapy were followed for ten years. Those consuming antioxidants did not require drug therapy with L-dopa as early in the illness as those who received no antioxidants. The doctors conducting this trial concluded that, "the progression of Parkinson's disease may be slowed by administration of these antioxidants."[15]

A common complication of diabetes is damage to nerves resulting in pain, numbness, and tingling—a condition called diabetic neuropathy. Damage to the retina leading to blindness also commonly occurs in diabetes. Diabetics have high levels of lipid peroxides in their bodies, a sign of free radical stress. Thus, using antioxidants may prove useful in protecting the nerves of diabetics from damage. In 1995, doctors gave diabetic patients with neuropathy 300 mg of the antioxidant lipoic acid twice each day. In as little as three weeks, there was a significant reduction in pain and numbness.[16]

Nerves on Fire

In the medical journal *The Lancet*, a nine-year-old boy was reported to suffer from a nervous system disease his doctors struggled to understand. At birth the boy appeared to be normal, but by age two he had such poor muscle tone he was confined to a wheelchair. Specialized testing finally revealed that he had a defect in one of the enzymes that mitochondria use to produce energy. As a result, high concentrations of free radicals damaged the boy's nervous system and muscular system. It was as though the sparks were flying and his nerves were on fire.

Doctors treating the boy thought the only way they could help him was to protect his nerve membranes by giving very high doses of antioxidants. They prescribed 2,000 IU of vitamin E per day, which is a tremendous dose, the RDA being only 8–10 IU per day. After several weeks of supplementation, the ATP (energy) level of his muscle had improved significantly. It was evidence that he was producing fewer damaging free radicals via his energy pathway. Remarkably, after vitamin E therapy he was able to walk for the first time.[17]

Reports such as these provide glimpses into what may be possible in the realm of treatment. They also provide strong incentive to make sure that the antioxidant defense system is richly supplied with the needed raw materials from the diet.

ANTIOXIDANT PROTECTION OF THE BRAIN FATTY ACIDS

It has become clear that in order to have an antioxidant defense system that works well, one must provide a complex of antioxidants rather than just one or two. Below is a list of antioxidants and their suggested range of intake for adults.

Suggested Ranges of Supplemental Antioxidants

Vitamin E	100-800 IU
Vitamin C	500-2,000 mg
Natural carotenes	10-300 mg
Glutathione	50-250 mg
Lipoic acid	25-50 mg
Coenzyme Q10	30-100 mg
Riboflavin (B2)	10-50 mg
Proanthocyanadins	25-100 mg
Mixed bioflavonoids	100-1,000 mg
Zinc	10-25 mg
Copper	1-3 mg
Selenium	25-50 mcg
Manganese	2-10 mg

Vitamin E is among the most important of the fat-soluble antioxidants. It is perfect for the fatty cell layers of the neuron membrane. Vitamin E sits nestled among the various phospholipid, fatty acid, and cholesterol molecules (Figure 11). When a rogue electron, chemical, or free-radical substance threatens or damages one of the fatty acids, vitamin E immediately goes to work to "put out the fire." Were vitamin E to shirk its duty, or be unavailable for action, the rogue free radical might trigger a chain reaction in which *many* fatty acid molecules are damaged. This makes vitamin E a key sentinel in the nervous system.

The importance of vitamin E in the brain was highlighted in a paper entitled "Vitamin E Deficiency and Neurological Disease." In this paper, Ronald Sokol, M.D., reviews the many and varied nervous system symptoms that can occur as a result of vitamin E insufficiency. He remarks, "It is now clear that vitamin E is an essential nutrient necessary for the optimal development and maintenance of the integrity and function of the human nervous system."[18]

Vitamin E supplementation becomes especially important when the diet is high in essential fatty acids or when one supplements with essential fatty acids. This was made clear some years ago when increased fish oil intake was associated with depleted vi-

Figure 11
How Vitamin E May Protect Nerve Cells from Free Radical Attack

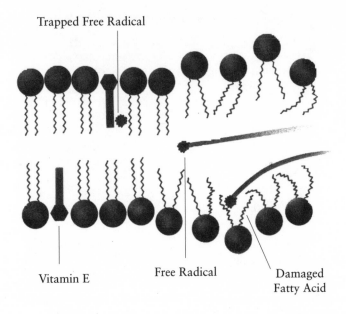

Trapped Free Radical

Vitamin E   Free Radical   Damaged
                                         Fatty Acid

Free radicals can damage nerve cell fatty acids and set up chain reactions in which hundreds of fatty acids may be damaged. This is somewhat like the spread of a wildfire. Vitamin E sits nestled in the nerve cell membrane to trap any rogue free radicals. When vitamin E (and other antioxidants) are in short supply, the delicate fatty acids of nerve cells are at risk to free radical attack.

tamin E and increased lipid peroxides in red blood cell membranes.[19] Therefore, whenever you increase your intake of unsaturated fatty acids you must increase your intake of vitamin E.

The form of vitamin E used in supplementation is important. The best form is d-alpha-tocopherol or a true mixed tocopherol. The true mixed tocopherol should also contain gamma-tocopherol, important in membranes, and tocotrienols. The synthetic form of vitamin E, dl-alpha-tocopherol, should not be used.

Antioxidant-Rich Foods[20]

Vitamin C

Food	Amount	Milligrams
Broccoli	1/2 cup	58.2
Brussels sprouts	1/2 cup	35.6
Cantaloupe	1/4 melon	56.4
Cauliflower	1/2 cup	34.3
Clams	1 pint	98.0
Currants, fresh	1/2 cup	101.4
Mango	1	53.7
Green Pepper	1	89.3
Hot pepper	1	46.2
Kiwi fruit	1	74.5
Papaya	1	187.8
Orange	1	131.0
Orange juice	6 oz.	155.0
Grapefruit	1/2 fruit	120.0
Grapefruit juice	6 oz.	185.0

Vitamin E

Food	Amount	International Units
Apricots, dried	1 cup	7.0
Mango	1	2.3
Olive oil	1/2 cup	12.9
Assorted nuts	1 cup	12.9
Pumpkin seeds	1/2 cup	2.5
Fortified cereals	1 cup	27.3
Sweet potato	1	5.8
Wheat germ	3.5 oz.	14.1
Sunflower seeds	3.5 oz.	44.0
Kale, raw	3.5 oz.	8.0

Beta-Carotene

Food	Amount	International Units
Broccoli	1/2 cup	1,082
Carrots, cooked	1/2 cup	19,152
Carrots, raw	1	20,253
Cereal grass	100 grams	10,000-50,000
Chlorella	100 grams	55,000
Dunaliella	100 grams	8,300,000
Sweet potato	1	21,822
Yellow squash	1/2 cup	3,628
Spinach, cooked	1/2 cup	7,371
Spinach, raw	1/2 cup	1,847
Tomato	1	766
Kale, cooked	1/2 cup	2,762
Cantaloupe	1/4 melon	4,304

PHYTONUTRIENTS THAT MAY PROTECT THE BRAIN AND NERVES

Beyond the commonly cited antioxidant nutrients, there are a number of other substances in plant foods that may protect the brain. Below is a sample list of some of the plant substances being used.

Food	Antioxidant	Proposed Action
Ginkgo biloba	Flavones, ginkgoflavonglycosides	Protect brain's blood supply
Green tea	Polyphenols (catechins)	Protect brain's blood supply
Bilberry	Anthocyanadins	Protect blood supply, eyes
Turmeric	Curcumins	Modifies inflammatory prostaglandins
Ginger	Phenylalkylketones	Modifies inflammatory prostaglandins
Citrus fruits	Quercitin	Modifies inflammatory prostaglandins
Grape seed	Proanthocyanadins	Protect vascular supply
Various fruits	Hesperidin	Prevents nerve oxidative stress

Recently, scientists at the USDA Human Nutrition Research Center on Aging at Tufts University measured the antioxidant activity of twenty-two common vegetables, one green tea, and one black tea. They measured the ability to protect against certain free radical substances including peroxyl radical and hydroxyl radical. The best of those tested are listed below.[21]

Best Protection Against Peroxyl Radical	Best Protection Against Hydroxyl Radical
Green, black tea	Kale
Garlic	Brussels sprouts
Kale	Alfalfa sprouts
Spinach	Beets
Brussels sprouts	Spinach
Alfalfa sprouts	Broccoli flowers
Beets	Red and bell pepper
Red and bell pepper	

In my opinion, the best way to increase brain-protecting phytonutrients is to increase consumption of whole fruits, vegetables, and herbs. Juicing with one of the excellent commercial juicers available is a convenient and efficient way to enrich your diet with the thousands of phytonutrients found in plants.

CAN THE BRAIN GO RANCID?

While there is much to learn, I think the evidence shows that the brain can go rancid. Keep in mind that I am not talking about the entire brain going rancid (being damaged by lipid peroxides). This would take a catastrophic event. I am referring to the fact that nerve cell membranes can suffer from lipid peroxidation. This damages nerves. Sometimes, clusters of brain tissue or entire regions suffer damage, which mildly or severely alters brain function.

How might we prevent this from occurring? I think it involves five basic features:

- Ensure the proper balance of fats and oils.
- Ensure the proper nutrients for efficient operation of the mitochondrial energy pathways.
- Ensure the proper balance of antioxidants to protect the mitochondria from their own intense activities.
- Ensure the proper balance of antioxidants to protect the nerve membranes from damage, regardless of the origin of the stress.
- Ensure proper function of the body's detoxication system and minimize exposure to toxins.

Numbers three and four share considerable overlap. However, there are subtle qualities that make their needs unique. Number five is beyond the scope of this discussion. However, proper essential fatty acid balance is also necessary for optimal function of the detoxication system. In general, all five of these can be achieved through smart nutritional practices.

Always remember, however, whenever you increase the intake of essential fatty acids, **you must increase your intake of**

antioxidant nutrients. In doing so, you must increase the full complement of antioxidants, not just one or two.

Even though you may have done all of the above, there is still a question that must be answered. What is the consequence of eating fats that are altered before you put them in your mouth? In the next chapter, we will explore a nemesis lurking in the diet—the trans fatty acids.

CHAPTER 7

THE FRENCH FRY GENERATION: AVOIDING THE HARMFUL BRAIN FATS

If you've ever stood at the fast food counter you may well remember the aroma of french fries as it flooded the air. Or perhaps you have stood at the doughnut counter, imbibing the sweet aroma of doughnuts as it wafted its way through your senses. As you readied to fill your body with these staples of American cuisine, you probably gave no thought to the bubbling sea of brown in which your fries or doughnuts were prepared. You probably gave little thought to the fate of the bubbling oils or to their fate once they entered your body. But should you think about it? If the brain is partially composed of diet-derived fat, should we wonder about the peculiar fats that give our french fries and doughnuts their flavor?

Taken a step further, should we wonder about deep-fried chicken nuggets, deep-fried mushrooms, deep-fried cheese balls, the fish burgers, and potato chips? All are rich with damaged oils. And, what about margarine? It's not deep-fried, but it's full of altered fats.

THE HARMFUL FATS: TRANS FATTY ACIDS AND THE BRAIN

Foods like those mentioned above are full of altered fats called *trans* fatty acids. Trans fatty acids occur when any unsaturated oil is heated for long periods, as in deep frying. They also form from

85

hydrogenation processes used in making margarine, shortening, and other products. Anything, therefore, that contains partially hydrogenated fat contains trans fatty acids. Deep-fried foods contain an abundance of trans fatty acids as do many packaged and prepared foods.

Normal fatty acids exist in what is known as the *cis* configuration. Cis means literally "on the same side." These fatty acids have their hydrogens on the same side wherever there is a double bond. As a result, their shape tends to be curved and becomes more curved with increasing double bonds. Brain fats like DHA have six double bonds and are curved in shape, vital to maintaining the electrical properties of nerve cell membranes.

Trans means "on the other side." In a trans fatty acid, the hydrogens have flipped to opposite sides of the double bond. This makes the fatty acid more straight, or arrow-shaped. With this change in shape comes a change in the way they behave in the cell membrane. They tend to be solid at body temperature and act more like saturated fat. Thus, trans fats make cell membranes more rigid and inflexible. They interfere with the normal functional properties of the cell membrane. Trans fatty acids are *not needed* in the brain and have none of the valuable properties of the brain-fats like DHA. Moreover, your body cannot make brain-fats like DHA from a trans fatty acid.

Dr. Donald Rudin refers to trans fatty acids as "funny fats," alluding to their peculiar shape and function. Though they are indeed "funny" one could argue that there is nothing funny about the way in which they influence the brain and body.

THE FLEXIBILITY FACTOR

In order to function properly, your brain cells (or any body cell) must have a certain degree of flexibility. This is maintained by having a balance of saturated fat, unsaturated fat, cholesterol, and other fats in the nerve cell membranes. It is the unsaturated fatty acids that give brain membranes their supple, fluid qualities. When you introduce trans fatty acids into the equation a whole range of new concerns emerges.

For example, scientists studying the width of the cis-form (normal form) of linoleic acid found it to be curved in shape and 11.3 angstroms wide. (Figure 12) This shape and size helps give cell membranes their fluid properties and appears to be needed to properly hold all of the various receptors in place. The same researchers showed the trans-form of linoleic acid to be only 3.2 angstroms wide. In simple terms, this means that the abnormal trans fatty acid occupies only one-fourth the space in the membrane of its normal cis-fatty acid counterpart.

Figure 12
The Shape of Things

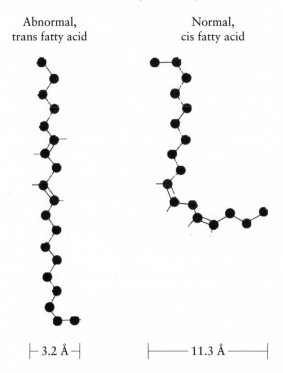

Abnormal,
trans fatty acid

Normal,
cis fatty acid

├─ 3.2 Å ─┤   ├──── 11.3 Å ────┤

Normal, cis fatty acids are curved, almost U-shaped molecules. Because of their expansive shape they make nerve membranes less densely packed and more flexible. Trans fatty acids are more straight and arrow shaped. They make nerve membranes more densely packed and rigid. Trans molecules are undesirable in the brain. Adapted from Simopoulos, AT. Trans Fatty Acids. In Spiller, GE, ed. Handbook of Lipids in Human Nutrition. Boca Raton, Florida: CRC Press, 1996:92.

Commenting on the different structure of trans fatty acids, Dr. R. S. Lees wrote that they are not only structurally similar to [saturated fat], but behave metabolically in an peculiar way.[1] If we are concerned about fat intake and the brain, the very striking difference in size and shape of the trans fatty acid should cause us to be very cautious.

DO TRANS FATTY ACIDS ENTER THE BRAIN?

It is now clear that trans fatty acids enter the body and become lodged within the cell membranes of various organs. The question of whether trans fatty acids enter the brain has recently been highlighted by some disturbing trends in the animal kingdom. In 1980, Dr. G. A. Dopeshwarkar showed that trans fatty acids readily crossed the placenta and ended up in almost every tissue in the offspring, including brain. When mothers continued consuming altered fats during the nursing period, trans fatty acids in the brain of their young became even more concentrated. And his most startling finding: he discovered that trans fatty acids, when taken into brain membranes, were inserted into the position where DHA normally resides.[2]

Writing in the journal *Lipids,* Dr. A. Grandgirard reported that trans fatty acids in the diet also showed up in the brains of animals. The brain tissues containing the highest levels were synaptosomes, retina, and tiny blood vessels called microvessels. Trans fatty acids were also found in myelin, the insulating sheath surrounding nerves, and in the sciatic nerve. He even noticed changes on an electrical measurement called an electroretinogram, which indicated the trans fats caused problems with vision.[3]

When intake of trans fatty acids was accompanied by low levels of the omega-3 alpha-linolenic acid, the uptake of trans fatty acids into the brain *doubled.* If the findings apply to humans this would be worrisome because intake of alpha-linolenic acid is already too low in affluent societies. Further, he found that when trans fatty acids in the diet were high, the brain fat DHA was replaced by a poor substitute called DPA.

In 1992, Dr. J. Petersen reported on his observations. He showed that when trans fatty acids were consumed they found their way into brain tissue as well as into the liver and heart. As dietary trans fatty acid levels increased, increasingly higher levels were found in tissues. Petersen, like Dr. Grandgirard, also found that "dietary trans fatty acids increased the percentage of DPA in the brain."[4]

THE IMPLICATIONS OF TRANS FATS IN THE BRAIN

These observations represent only a portion of those that have been reported. We cannot always extend our observations of animals to humans; however, much of the other brain fatty acid findings have proven true for humans as well as animals. There is concern about the potential dangers that exist for the human brain. This is especially true since *there is absolutely no nutritional value gained from eating trans fatty acids*. Hence, we have only potential risk.

Two additional factors deserve our consideration. We are a culture that consumes very low amounts of brain-fats such as DHA (and its parent alpha-linolenic acid). This creates a potential problem that may affect brain structure and function. Moreover, high intake of saturated fat coupled with the high intake of trans fatty acids cause the potential problems to multiply. The margin for error grows smaller. The expression of any genetic weakness grows more likely.

Adequate intake of unsaturated fatty acids like DHA and ALA can help minimize the chance that trans fatty acids will be taken up by our brain and nerves. Unfortunately, trans fatty acids can block the enzymes needed to manufacture our own DHA.

BLOCKING YOUR OWN BRAIN FATS

Recall from Chapter Four that there are two ways we can get DHA for the brain. We can get it directly from our food or we can make it from the omega-3 essential fatty acid alpha-linolenic acid.

When we do not obtain enough DHA through the diet, as is true of many people, we begin to rely more heavily on our ability to make our own DHA. Thus, ability to change alpha-linolenic acid to DHA becomes more vital.

Here is where the problem lies. Several studies have shown that trans fatty acids impair our ability to do this. In essence, you may further compromise your brain by limiting the synthesis of your most critical neural fatty acid, DHA.[5,6] Thus, not only do we have concerns about how trans fatty acids might be directly taken up into the brain, but also how they may interfere with the manufacture of our own brain fats.

This point was emphasized by Dr. Dopeshwarkar who stated, "In the case of borderline EFA [essential fatty acid] deficiency this suppression by trans fatty acids may aggravate EFA deficiency and its consequences on brain metabolism."[7] On the same topic, Dr. Ralph Holman, who has worked in collaboration with Mayo Clinic researchers, concluded: "Large scale hydrogenation of vegetable oils reduces omega-3 and omega-6 fatty acids and replaces them by saturated and [trans fatty acids] that interfere with the omega-3 and omega-6 metabolism, inducing significant partial deficiencies of essential fatty acids." He further stated that, "It would seem wise to avoid foods that contain unusual or unnatural [fatty acids]."[8]

OUT OF THE FLOW

From above, there are two ways that trans fatty acids might harm the brain. They may be taken up directly into nerve membranes and they may block your body's ability to make its own brain-fat DHA. There also appears to be a third way they can influence your brain. In Chapter Three, I discussed how important the blood supply is to maintaining peak brain power. Consuming trans fatty acids may also affect your brain's blood supply.

Scientists have learned that trans fatty acids appear to increase the "bad" form of cholesterol (LDL), they decrease the "good" form (HDL), they increase triglycerides, and they increase Lp(a) (lipoprotein a). Lp(a) is a protein that contributes to plaque in

blood vessels, atherosclerosis, and blood clots. Elevated triglycerides, as we saw in Chapter Three, may contribute to blood
sludging, which reduces the oxygen supply to the brain. In this
way, trans fatty acids might be one of the food factors that slows
the blood supply to the brain or increase your risk to stroke.[9]

TRANS FATTY ACIDS IN THE DIET

How common are trans fatty acids in the diet and where do we get
them? Dr. Mary Enig has studied the trans fatty acid content of
foods for some two decades and has noticed some disturbing
trends. When she looked at the trans fat content of a *small* bag of
snack chips it contained over twenty-five percent of its fat as trans
fatty acids. (Below one percent is ideal.)

This was true of eight out of ten different brands. The highest
level found was forty-seven percent trans. Imagine, almost half of
the fat in a bag of chips may occur as trans fatty acids. The total
amount of trans fat in one of these bags was up to 4.6 grams, or
almost a teaspoon. A serving of french fries fried in vegetable oil
contained up to 8.2 grams of trans fatty acids. Deep-fried fish fil-
lets contained up to 8.0 grams of trans fats. A single doughnut
contained almost 13 grams of trans fatty acids.[10]

Estimates by Dr. Enig suggest that the total fat intake of an
American man ranges from 145 to 258 grams per day. A woman's
average is slightly less. If roughly twenty-five percent of this fat
comes from trans fatty acids, approximately 38 grams of trans
fatty acids might be consumed daily (as an upper limit). This is an
astonishing amount if Dr. Enig is correct. If trans fats do indeed
find their way into the brain, trans fats may be a significant factor
in declining brain power for some people.

A MESSAGE FOR MOTHERS AND INFANTS:
TRANS FATTY ACIDS IN BREAST MILK

Exposure to trans fatty acids can occur very early in life. Surprisingly, breastmilk and infant formula can be the first trans fat-con-

taining foods to which a child is exposed. According to one study, trans fatty acids increase in the blood of nursing infants between two and eight weeks after birth. At two months, the level is almost twice as high in breast-fed babies as in formula-fed babies.[11]

Bolstering this idea is the work of Canadian doctors who measured trans fatty acids in the breast milk of 198 mothers. They found the range of trans fatty acids in breast milk was up to twenty percent of total fat. Upon careful analysis, the researchers concluded that about ninety percent of Canadian lactating women have moderate to high levels of trans fatty acids in their breast milk.

How do such high levels of trans fatty acids find their way into mother's milk? Diet is the most likely source. Using mathematical calculations based on other data, it was estimated that women who had high levels of trans fatty acids in their breast milk consumed diets in which about twenty-six percent of their fat came from trans fatty acids. The women considered to be in the moderate trans fatty acid group consumed about 10 grams of trans fatty acids per day.

Dr. Chen and his colleagues remarked on the high trans fats in breast milk. They stated, "It is clear that trans fatty acid[s] present in partially hydrogenated vegetable oils are transferred to human milk through maternal diets and, subsequently, to infants." They also noticed that as trans fatty acid levels increased in breastmilk the level of omega-3 alpha-linolenic acid decreased. They continued, "the elevation of trans fatty acids in human milk is at the expense of linoleic acid and linolenic acid because the high trans products contain less [of these fatty acids]."[12] (It is also interesting to note that trans fatty acid levels are quite high in cow's milk.")[13]

Protecting Against Trans Fatty Acids in Breast Milk

Breast milk is still far superior to formula for infant development. To protect against excessive trans fatty acid in breast milk, mothers should:

- Restrict the dietary intake of trans fatty acids during conception, pregnancy, and lactation.

- Ensure that antioxidant nutrient levels are optimal.
- Ensure that omega-3 fatty acid levels in the diet are optimal, since they appear to lower the chance that dietary trans fatty acids will be taken up into brain.

A MESSAGE FOR TEENAGE GIRLS

The teenage years are a critical time for young girls because this is a time of rapid change, growth, and development. It is also the time that young girls are able to have children. There is convincing evidence that the adolescent years may be one of the most critical periods for protecting the brain of a developing child. Nutritional status during pregnancy is important, but the period before conception is critical as well.

Dr. Michael Crawford, of the Institute of Brain Biochemistry and Human Nutrition in London, has studied the fatty acid intakes of humans of various ages, as well as animals, from around the globe. He emphasizes the importance of preconception nutrition and states, "It is not just what the mother eats while she is pregnant but her background nutrition which prepares her, possibly during and from puberty."[14] Crawford and others have begun to recognize that the nutritional status of adolescent girls is extremely important to the development of the brains of their children, even though they may not bear a child for some years after adolescence.

This brings up the issue of trans fatty acids. In the analysis of trans fatty acids performed on teenage girls, up to fifteen percent of the fats consumed were trans fatty acids. The daily average was three grams, but ranged up to eight grams. The source of trans fatty acids was most commonly cookies, cakes, bread, rolls, and crackers; foods often prepared with partially hydrogenated oils.[15]

A MESSAGE FOR ADULTS: THE EFFECT OF TRANS FATTY ACIDS

The findings on breast milk and infant trans fatty acids is very important for these critical periods. But what is the relevance to adults? Recall from above that trans fatty acids impair the enzymes we need to convert dietary fatty acids into the brain-fats and messengers. These enzymes normally tire out as we age, so anything that might further slow their activity would not be conducive to peak brain power. Trans fats also increase triglycerides, which can contribute to blood sludging. They increase lipoprotein a, which may contribute to plaque formation in the brain's blood vessels.[16]

Consider also that you are very likely part of a generation that was raised on junk food and snacks that contained large amounts of trans fatty acids. You may have been consuming trans fatty acids for some twenty or thirty years or more. You are also likely part of a generation raised on a low intake of DHA and ALA. You were perhaps bottle fed and, thus, *received no DHA in your first six months or life or longer*—a period of rapid brain formation. These two factors alone have been shown to be ingredients for rapid uptake of trans fats into the brain.

As you approach your thirties, forties, fifties, sixties, or seventies you may be growing concerned about problems of memory. You may be concerned about disorders of mood and behavior. You may be concerned about friends, a family member, or yourself developing a neurological disease. You may be concerned about risk of stroke.

It is my opinion that the intake of trans fatty acids has important implications for adults. I think it becomes more important with each passing generation because the brain consequences of inadequate fatty acids seems to grow larger with each generation raised on inadequate diets. (See Chapter Fourteen.) Only time and additional research will tell us for certain. But I'm willing to err on the side of caution and restrict foods that contain trans fatty acids. The risk of doing so is almost nil. The potential benefits are significant.

WHO SHOULD AVOID TRANS FATTY ACIDS?

There is a wide range of common foods in the diet that contain trans fatty acids. I used to think that as long as one consumed a diet of healthy fats that is rich in nutrients, occasional consumption of trans fatty acids was not a serious breach. As we discover more about trans fatty acids and how they might influence the brain, there appears to be no good reason why anyone would knowingly consume trans fat-containing foods. While everyone may benefit from reducing intake of trans fatty acids, there are some special circumstances in which more strict avoidance is crucial.

Pregnant and Nursing Mothers

Pregnant and nursing mothers should treat trans fatty acid-containing foods as they would treat any harmful substance. Avoid them, remembering that the architecture of the baby's brain may be negatively influenced. Women anticipating having a baby should avoid trans fatty acids for as long as they can before conception. The same is true for men. (Remember that even sperm have a high requirement for long-chain fatty acids like DHA.)

Brain and Nervous System Diseases

Individuals with neurological diseases such as multiple sclerosis, Alzheimer's, Parkinson's, ALS, and others should avoid trans fats. While there is yet no definitive proof that trans fats aggravate these conditions, I believe any practice that might restore the fatty portion of brain architecture is important to pursue.

Heart and Blood Vessel Disorders

People with a family history of heart disease, atherosclerosis, or stroke should avoid eating trans fatty acids. These fats do all the wrong things needed for blood fats and they may eventually affect the brain's blood supply.

Learning, Mood, and Behavioral Disorders

Those who suffer from behavioral disorders such as attention deficit, hyperactivity, depression, schizophrenia, and postpartum depression should also avoid trans fats. In the following chapters, I build a correlation between neural fatty acids and these conditions. Since trans fatty acids modify neural fatty acids to an unknown extent, I think it is wise to avoid them when suffering from these conditions.

Toddlers and Small Children

Toddlers and small children should avoid trans fatty acids as a matter of family policy. During this period of life, the brain is developing rapidly. New connections are being made, myelin is being formed to insulate nerve fibers, the brain is increasing in size, the future is being established. To expose children at this age to trans fatty acids is doing them a considerable disservice.

Adulthood and Aging

Aging individuals who are concerned about declining mental faculties should perhaps avoid trans fatty acids. We will see in later chapters that taking certain fatty acid substances may improve the age-related decline in memory and thinking that is so common as one ages. One can infer from such studies that improving neural membranes is, therefore, important to such function. In this regard, decreasing the dietary intake of trans fatty acids would be of benefit to the membranes of the aging brain.

Peak Mental Performance

I believe the role of fatty acids in brain function is so important that anyone who wants to achieve peak mental performance could benefit from avoiding trans fats. Sure, we can all probably cite examples of a genius in our work, college, or high school class who pumped down bags of chips and fries and managed to outperform the rest of us. How is it that the diets of these people did not impair their performance? It is a legitimate question. I wonder, however, to what heights such people may have risen had they eaten foods that fostered better brain power. We don't have absolute proof that avoiding trans fatty acids will improve your mental function. The weight of evidence, however, has convinced me that fatty acid balance matters in the long run. I'll take my chances on a clean diet without being fanatical about it.

THE TRANS-FREE DIET

When we look at foods that contain trans fatty acids, it becomes clear that many of life's delectable pleasures are on the list. It is sad, but true. However, remember that fat is critical to our very existence. This is likely why our taste buds have developed such an affinity for fatty foods. Now, our ability to manipulate fats in food has made us prisoners to our fat cravings. We are led by our taste buds to fats that no longer serve our survival needs. In fact, they may even threaten them.

Below is a list to help you gauge your intake of trans fatty acids. It shows the most common foods known to contain high amounts of trans fatty acids:

French fries	Deep fried fish burgers
Candy	Deep fried mushrooms, cheese curds, etc.
Potato chips	Puffed cheese snacks
Corn chips	Tortilla chips
Cookies	Deep fried chicken nuggets
Cake	Doughnuts
Mayonnaise	Margarine
Shortening	Salad dressing (other than olive oil-based)

Anything that contains one or all of the following on its label probably contains trans fatty acids: "*may contain partially hydrogenated* soybean oil, sunflower oil, safflower oil, or corn oil." Minimize these foods. If some of the items on the above list say "baked" on the label, they are probably not deep-fried in oil. Baked fries are a better choice, but be alert to the kind of oil used on the chips. In general, baked corn chips tend to have less trans fatty acids than most other corn chips.

Many salad dressings contain high levels of trans fatty acids. This presents a difficulty for the person who wants to have healthy salad. The best choice of dressing is probably a vinegar and oil dressing where olive oil is used. Olive oil is high in the omega-9 fatty acid oleic acid, which only has one double bond. It is, thus, very stable and does not easily form trans fatty acids. Hazelnut oil is also a good salad oil choice. Canola oil provides a nice oil for salads, but it should be mixed on the eve of use because of its modest omega-3 content.

REMOVING TRANS FATTY ACIDS FROM THE BODY

While our diets and bodies have been overburdened with trans fatty acids, there is a strategy that can begin to reverse the tide. This is based on the fortunate fact that our cells are replaced on a regular basis. By getting trans fats out of the diet and supplying ample amounts of essential fatty acids we gradually replace the membrane fatty acids as new membranes are made. If you provide a good balance of fatty acids this transformation is positive. If you continue to supply trans fatty acids, you gain little ground.

Reducing your cell burden of trans fatty acids generally means consuming daily amounts of omega-3-rich oils. In Chapter Twelve, I describe the fats and oils needed in a *Smart-Fat Diet*. By switching to these oils we can begin the process of ridding our bodies of accumulated trans fatty acids and restore our membranes to their supple, soft, and fluid natural state.

CHAPTER 8

THE WINDOW OF TIME: CRITICAL PERIODS THROUGHOUT LIFE

Jean was seven months pregnant when she decided to complete a long-overdue home landscaping project. She spent almost an entire day shoveling white rock and pushing a wheelbarrow across a bumpy lawn—a task made more difficult by a protruding abdomen and the added weight of a developing child. The next morning, Jean awoke with a terrible lower-back ache, but went to work nonetheless. As the day wore on, her excruciating back pain worsened. Rather than go home she took couple of aspirin, hoping the pain was the mere aftermath of her weekend with the shovel. Within ten minutes, her placenta tore and she began bleeding heavily. Jean went into labor and was rushed to the hospital—labor pains just two minutes apart.

She spent four days in the hospital as doctors brought her condition under control. Her physicians were concerned about a delivery so early in the pregnancy. Should she give birth now, the baby would face a long, uphill battle in its first months of life; perhaps throughout its lifetime. The doctors wanted to prevent the baby from delivering for as long as possible, but only managed to delay the birth another two weeks. Stacy was born six weeks premature and weighed only five pounds.

At the four month check-up, her doctor noticed that her feet would not bend downward at the ankle. Stacy was not yet rolling and was not as mobile as a normal child her age. As Stacy grew her movement problems became more evident and learning problems became obvious. She was continually behind her peers in school.

In Stacy's case, the torn placenta quite likely interrupted oxygen flow to the brain. This alone might be cause for her neurological problems. However, because she was premature, she may not have received adequate brain-fats a normal child might receive from the placenta when carried to full term. These fats were never replaced as she grew, so the fatty acid problem within the brain was never corrected and, perhaps, even worsened.

Stacy's outcome is more happy than many such children. She began taking DHA at a dose of about 200 mg per day. After eight months on this regimen, her movement problems improved and her learning problems showed striking improvement.[1]

Throughout life, there are various periods in which the brain is highly sensitive to the kinds of fats and oils it receives. If appropriate fats and oils are not supplied during these periods, the brain structures developing at that time may not form properly, or may become susceptible to damage. Most doctors agree that pregnancy and infancy are critical periods, but according to William E. Connor, M.D., of the Department of Medicine at Oregon Health Sciences University, "In all probability, requirements for n-3 fatty acids continue during childhood and even in adult life. There should be adequate amounts of n-3 and n-6 fatty acids in the diet throughout life and their ratio is of great importance."[2]

Below is a list of periods during which fatty acid balance is critical. At first glance, it becomes evident that almost all of life's periods are represented here. This reflects our growing understanding of the importance of fatty acid balance in all stages of life.

- Pregnancy (effects on woman)
- Women during childbearing years
- Fetal period (effects on developing child)
- Infancy
- Childhood including adolescence
- Adulthood

If we meet these critical periods with the best possible balance of essential fatty acids we may set the stage for a bright and healthy future. If we do not meet these critical periods, there may be consequences that last throughout life. A brief look at each of these periods will show the importance of establishing and maintaining proper fatty acid balance.

PREGNANT MOTHERS: EFFECTS ON MOTHER AND CHILD

Doctors have been surprised to discover that, during pregnancy, the blood levels of key neural fatty acids appear to drop dramatically. This probably occurs as a result of the developing child's demand for neural fatty acids. The fetal brain develops rapidly throughout pregnancy and its demand for long-chain fatty acids like arachidonic acid and DHA can only be met by the mother. To achieve adequate levels for brain development, the baby essentially robs the mother of these fatty acids by taking them from the placental blood.

In order for an unborn child to develop properly, the mother must replenish her stores of DHA and arachidonic acid (AA) so that she is able to continue supplying these vital nutrients to the fetus throughout the pregnancy. Unfortunately, many mothers may have insufficient neural fatty acids in their own bodies and, thus, provide less than optimal amounts to their developing child. Vegetarian mothers must be especially aware of this fact.

This was made clear when doctors examined the fatty acid status of women in the third trimester of pregnancy and discovered an imbalance of omega-6 and omega-3 fatty acids in all cases. Omega-3 fatty acids such as alpha-linolenic acid (ALA) and DHA were found to be low, while the omega-6 linoleic acid was too high. This probably happened because they ate too much oil that contained omega-6 fatty acids such as linoleic acid and consumed too few foods containing omega-3 fatty acids.

The authors concluded that these changes "have serious consequences for the developing fetus since a reduced level of omega-3 fatty acids can affect learning, behavioral, visual, and retinal function in low birth weight infants. Pregnancy may result in essential fatty acid deficiency as a result of physiologic stress. Pregnant women's diets should be modified to contain less linoleic acid and more alpha-linolenic acid so the manufacture of long-chain polyunsaturated fatty acids [DHA] is optimized. Mothers should consume fatty fish regularly so that they get adequate amounts of DHA."[3]

Dr. Ralph Holman, of the University of Minnesota, has also measured the blood fatty acids of women during normal pregnancies. Holman's group found that during pregnancy, the level of omega-3 fatty acids fell considerably when compared with non-pregnant women. The abnormal fatty acid profiles persisted for at least six weeks after delivery, at which time the study was terminated. It is possible that fatty acid inadequacy may have persisted much longer than six weeks postpartum.[4]

In Dr. Holman's study, DHA was the most depressed being found at only thirty-five percent of its prepregnancy level. ALA, EPA, and DHA all further decreased during the postpartum period. His work suggests that during pregnancy the omega-3 fatty acid levels fall significantly and that low levels continue to persist after delivery.

Dr. Holman strongly emphasizes that the requirements for omega-3 fatty acids are highest during the development of the fetal nervous system, which is rich in these fats. He appears to recommend supplementation with DHA when he states, "Because essential fatty acids decrease in the maternal circulation during pregnancy and remain low at least six weeks beyond the pregnancy, it may be reasonable to increase the omega-3 polyunsaturated fatty acids in the diet before, during, and after pregnancy."[5]

WOMEN OF CHILDBEARING AGE: EFFECTS ON HEALTH AND WELLBEING

There are two reasons for women of childbearing age to pay close attention to dietary fat balance. First, because their fatty acid status will determine the fats available to the developing brain of their child or children. This becomes important well before conception of a child. Second, pregnancy places such great demands on a mother's fatty acid stores that some women of childbearing age may suffer the personal consequences for years to come.

In a study similar to that of Dr. Holman, Dr. Monique Al and her colleagues studied long-chain fatty acids such as DHA in pregnant women. Her group found that the mother's DHA stores declined during pregnancy and that they became worse with each one. Dr. Al's group concluded, "during pregnancy, maternal DHA is mobilized from a store that is not easily replenished after delivery. As a result, the maternal and neonatal [infant] DHA status diminishes with each subsequent pregnancy."[6]

Dr. Al's comments about DHA status declining further with each subsequent pregnancy is important. This phenomenon may be linked, in part, to the high rates of depression in women compared with men. Moreover, there are other disorders of adult women such as PMS that are associated with abnormal fatty acid levels. Chronic fatigue and chronic fatigue syndrome, which more often affect women, have also been found to be associated with abnormal fatty acid levels. Multiple sclerosis is more common among women and has been associated with fatty acid abnormalities.

The findings of Dr. Al and others may mean that women who have had children, even though they may not currently be pregnant, might need fatty acid supplementation to restore their depleted reserves. Adult women wishing to become pregnant should also ensure that their fatty acid status is at its peak.

While many of these studies focused on DHA, I believe that many doctors will agree that achieving a balance between GLA, ALA, DHA, and AA in adult women and during pregnancy is important. This can be achieved by supplemental doses of fish oil, DHA-rich oil, GLA-rich primrose oil, and ALA-rich flax seed oil. Since each pregnancy is unique and we are usually careful about supplementation during pregnancy, it may be wise to consult a health care professional to establish the right amounts for a given individual. This is especially true if the mother has a neurological disorder such as MS or seizures.

GROWING A NEW BRAIN: THE FETAL PERIOD

During gestation, the fetal brain may grow as many as 250,000 nerve cells each minute and will eventually manufacture on the order of 100 billion neurons. A remarkable seventy percent of the total brain cells that will last our lifetime have divided before birth. At six weeks, the growing brain of an embryo is almost as big as its body. By the third month of gestation, the brain is consuming about seventy percent of the energy delivered to the fetus. All of these activities demand a constant and very specific nutrient supply. With such a dramatic number of new cells being made each day the balance of brain fatty acids is crucial.

The work of Dr. Ralph Holman on essential fatty acids and fetal brain development perhaps sums it up best. He points out that:[7]

- The mental apparatus of the coming generation is developed in utero (during the fetal period).
- The time to begin supplementation with essential fatty acids is *before* conception.
- The normal brain *cannot* be made without omega-3 fatty acids, particularly DHA.
- There may be no later opportunity to repair effects of omega-3 fatty acid insufficiency once the nervous system is formed.

I believe Dr. Holman's comment that the normal brain cannot be made without omega-3 fatty acids should be emphasized. The story of premature babies strongly emphasizes this point and provides a lesson about all babies. Under normal circumstances, a child developing in the uterus receives its neural fatty acids from the mother's placenta. If the child is born prematurely, this supply of neural fatty acids is abruptly interrupted at a time when the brain has a critical need. In order to continue the normal brain development, the premature infant must receive these fatty acids from breast milk or formula.

Dr. Michael Crawford comments, "There is now evidence from several laboratories and our own that the premature infant is denied the substantial supply of AA and DHA that it otherwise would have received if it had remained as a fetus fed by the placenta. Within three to six days of birth, their concentrations [of neural fatty acids] may fall to less than one-fifth of those found in the placental-fetal blood supply."[8]

Prematurity is associated with all kinds of potential medical problems throughout life. It is very important that fatty acid needs be addressed in this age. If you have a child who is, for example, five years old, but was born prematurely, it may be that his or her neural fatty acid stores are not adequate and that he or she may benefit from supplementation and dietary changes. I would be especially suspicious in a child with learning, behavioral, or developmental problems who was born prematurely.

The Early Entry and Near Exit of Laura

Laura was born during the twenty-first week of gestation. This tiny, almost fetus-like infant no larger than the palm of an adult hand, spent the first weeks of her existence clinging to life inside an incubator. Despite heroic care and sophisticated medical intervention, she was not expected to live. Her tiny, frail body was almost translucent as she lay nearly motionless in her plastic bubble. Laura's mother Sarah was desperate for help and learned of Patricia Kane, Ph.D., a nutritional biochemist who has worked extensively with fatty acids and brain chemistry.

Sarah's diet was too low in essential fatty acids. Her breast milk was very low in fat, a fact made evident when the milk sat in its refrigerated storage. Dr. Kane's strategy was to feed substantial amounts of saturated and unsaturated fatty acids to Sarah so that her breast milk fatty acid content would rise to a level that would begin the regenerative process in her baby. The milk would then be fed through the feeding tube inserted into little Laura.

Within two weeks, the baby began to undergo a remarkable transformation. She was seen batting at a tiny star hanging inside the incubator using a surprising degree of eye-hand coordination for such a small infant. The nurse in attendance remarked that "In twenty-five years of nursing I have never seen any child of this age with such eye-hand coordination."

Laura's progress from this point was exceptional and she was taken home one month early. However, she still weighed only four pounds. While at home, she received further doses of essential fatty acids. During the ensuing months, Laura made periodic visits to her pediatrician who proclaimed her healthy. At age twenty months, Laura was taken back for a thorough evaluation by the director of the neonatal unit who was moved to tears by her progress. Rarely had a premature baby, especially one this premature, fared so well and been so healthy. Most developed cerebral palsy, severe visual problems, mental retardation, or other serious problems. Laura's journey to wholeness stands out as a victory of grand proportion and serves to further educate us about the power of fats and oils. Today, she is six years old and lives life as a perfectly normal child.

A Future Full of Promise

The fetal period is crucial to formation of the child's brain. It is a critical window in which over seventy percent of the brain's neurons will form. Echoing the sentiments of Dr. Holman, this may be the time during which we can ensure the best possible future for a child and allow him or her to realize the greatest potential.

THE INFANT PERIOD: WIRING FOR POTENTIAL

At birth, a baby's brain contains 100 billion neurons, roughly as many nerve cells as there are stars in the Milky Way. The infant brain grows rapidly during the first year of life. At birth, it weighs roughly 350 grams. By the end of the first year, it has nearly tripled in size, reaching a weight of over 1,000 grams. It achieves this phenomenal growth rate by 1) growth of existing nerve cells, 2) insulating nerves with myelin, 3) formation of branches, 4) and formation of synapses. Each nerve cell may form connections that number ten to twenty thousand. During this time, supportive cells called glial cells also increase into the trillions. This is especially true during the first six months of life.

During the first year, the "hard-wiring" process for such things as vision, feelings, movement, and language is a high priority. The foundation for mental, physical, and emotional intelligence is formed during this period and continues for many years. Infancy is a critical window of time, for if the neurons are not properly formed and connections are improperly made, the effects can haunt a child for his or her lifetime. When the foundation of the brain's architecture is properly in place, it can set the stage for a future filled with potential.

During the first year of life, the brain still demands an astonishing sixty percent of the total energy taken in by the infant. Most of this energy is used to form the myelin sheath around nerves and to manufacture nerve cell membranes.[10] If you recall our discussion from Chapter Two, each of these steps in brain-building requires fatty acids from the diet. One fatty acid in particular, DHA, is needed in especially high amounts since the infant *cannot make this fatty acid efficiently.* Because of the fatty acid demands of the rapidly growing infant brain, about fifty percent of the infant's calories *must* come from fat. This is compared with the adult where only about twenty to thirty percent of calories need to come from fat.

Feeding the Infant Brain: Breast milk and Brain Power

Breast milk is the finest form of nutrition for a developing infant's brain. It contains a diverse array of fatty acids including ALA, GLA, AA, and DHA. Breast-fed infants, when compared to formula-fed infants, appear to develop better visual acuity, higher IQ, and perhaps may even be protected against brain disorders later in life.[11,12,13] Even though breast milk is superior to formula, many breast-fed infants may be getting inadequate amounts of neural fatty acids.

In previous chapters, I described the omega-6 to omega-3 ratio. Recall that the ratio in today's diets ranges from 20 to 30:1.[14]

This is far too high when you remember the ideal ratio of 1:1. However, in breast milk the ratio has been found to range from 8:1 to a startling 45:1.[15]

Why would the mother's fatty acid levels vary so greatly? Most likely it reflects the wide variation of fatty acids in the diets of mothers. When we review studies on fatty acids in brain function, we must keep in mind that many breast fed babies in the West may still be receiving inadequate amounts of fatty acids because of the mother's meager intake. This is reflected in studies of the fatty acid ratios of different cultures. Below is a sample of the DHA levels found in breast milk of women of various countries. Notice the dramatic differences in DHA levels of Malaysia and India compared with the United States.

Breast Milk Content of DHA[16]

Country	DHA % of total fat
Malaysia	0.9
India	0.9
China	0.7
USA	0.3
Vegan	0.2

Another interesting cultural point is raised when we look at Inuit mothers from northern Quebec, Canada. Their diets are typically very high in seal blubber and other foods rich in omega-3 fatty acids. Unfortunately, the foods in their region are typically contaminated with organochlorine pesticides and PCBs. In fact, their breast milk contains four to seven times more of these toxins than non-Inuit mothers. Doctors expected to find brain degeneration and developmental delays in the children, but this has not been the case. This discovery has led doctors to suggest that omega-3 fatty acids may, at least partially, help protect the brain against toxic chemicals.[17]

Caution for Vegetarian Mothers

Vegetarian mothers must be especially aware that they get adequate DHA during pregnancy and while breast feeding, since vegans and vegetarians have been shown to have significantly lower DHA in breast milk. Their babies also show lower DHA. For example, Australian and British babies fed milk from omnivore mothers have about six percent DHA in the red blood cells. American infants have about three percent. British infants fed milk from vegetarian mothers have only two percent DHA in their red cells.[18] Using flax seed oil as a source of alpha-linolenic acid has been used by many vegetarian mothers in hopes of increasing their DHA levels. However, conversion of ALA to DHA appears to be insufficient for a pregnant or nursing mother.

Feeding the Infant Brain: Formula Inadequacy

Prior to 1998, infant formula contained no DHA. In many cases, formula also contained little or none of the other important long-chain fatty acids such as arachidonic acid. In addition to being low in unsaturated fatty acids, many formulas were derived from cow's milk, which is high in saturated fat. These differences in fatty acids may account for the fact that formula-fed infants tended to do worse on various types of visual, attention, and intelligence tests. Some formula manufacturers may rectify this particular problem before the year 2000 (though 24 countries, excluding the U.S., have already done so). The evidence below shows the price many children may have paid because of past formula inadequacy.

Neural Fatty Acids in the Brain: Formula vs. Breast Milk

For many years, doctors believed that the brain's structure was so vital that it was protected against dietary fluctuations. Studies comparing the brains of breast-fed infants and formula-fed infants reveal that dietary fatty acid intake in infants does indeed affect the brain's structure.

DHA Levels in Brain Tissue of Breast fed vs Bottle fed Infants[19]

Breast-Fed Infants	Formula-Fed Infants
phosphatidylserine, High DHA	Low DHA (DHA replaced by omega-6 fatty acids)
Phosphatidylethanolamine, High DHA	Low DHA (DHA replaced by omega-6 fatty acids, especially DPA)

Consequences of Low Brain DHA

What are the potential adverse effects of changing the fatty acid make-up of the brain? On this issue, the conclusion of Dr. J. Farquharson is of great concern. He states, "The reductions in the DHA content between the breast and artificially fed infants are of a magnitude that would be sufficient to *alter [brain] membrane function and could critically affect the resultant responses to electrical and chemical stimulation and alter membrane and neurotransmitter function.*"[emphasis added][20]

Farquharson believes these changes may contribute to degenerative disease of the nervous system later in life. He offers the opinion that "these short term effects and indeed the long term effects [of DHA inadequacy] on neuronal integrity that might predispose to adult neurodegenerative disease warrant urgent attention."

Building for the Future

While some of these findings may seem dire, they also suggest that providing proper fatty acid balance during the infant period raises the opportunity to ensure that any child can realize his or her peak potential. It also raises the very strong possibility that children suffering from learning, behavioral, or other brain-related problems, might be helped if fatty acid balance is restored while still a child. In addition, we perhaps have the chance to take this knowledge and give today's children the best opportunity of any generation in recent memory by attending to their critical brain nutrient needs early in life. To achieve this we must be sure that nursing mothers have adequate GLA, ALA, and DHA in their diets. We must also be certain that if formula is used that it contains these fatty acids as well.

GROWING BRIGHT AND STRONG: FATTY ACIDS IN CHILDREN

Beyond infancy, the brain continues to grow, forming new connections, myelinating fibers, forming new dendritic branches, and growing new glial cells. Many of the features most crucial to developing a healthy brain and nervous system must be honed and refined from ages one to ten. Development of speech, language, vocabulary, and visual acuity is firmly set in these years. Development of emotional health, fine motor control, and gross motor skills expand as life experience and stimulation of the brain continues. All of these processes are driven by the enriching experiences of a child's life.

In these early years, neural pathways are dedicated and formed based on the stimulating activities of childhood. Those that are not used and developed are pruned (or cut off) as the brain strives for efficiency of its connections. The brain's greatest growth spurt comes to a close around age ten. This is a period when the balance between forming nerve cells and destroying nerve cells comes to an end.

This window of ages one to ten is crucial to the foundation of the brain's structure. It will determine the extent and complexity of many of the brain's connections and will dramatically influence a child's future. The process of brain development continues to be influenced by the fatty acids that contribute to nerve-cell structure. It is during this phase of childhood that we cannot afford to overlook the very critical requirement of the brain for long-chain fatty acids.

Struggling with Jamie: A Lesson from Two Siblings

Jamie was a ten-year-old boy who seemed to struggle with behavioral problems almost from the beginning. He was inattentive, aggressive, and had difficulty with coordination. Sports were hard for him and learning was no better. What was very interesting about Jamie was that he was only ten months younger than his older brother Shane. Shane seemed to be bright, balanced, coordinated, and calm. One might have attributed Jamie's struggles to being the second child, but I think we overlook important biochemical clues with these assumptions.

Jamie also had patches of dry skin and coarse, unruly hair—clues to fatty acid imbalance. His mother's pregnancy was difficult. She also suffered from postpartum depression, which had to be treated with antidepressants. I was suspicious that perhaps his mother's fatty acid levels had not recovered from the first pregnancy and that Jamie was the unfortunate recipient of low brain fat levels while he was in the womb. This certainly fits with the research and also fits with what many doctors have observed with closely-spaced births. Quite often, the second child in closely-spaced births struggles because the nutritional demands of the prior pregnancy left the mother's reserves depleted.

Jamie began taking a balanced fatty acid supplement that contained DHA, GLA, and ALA from DHA oil, primrose oil, and flax seed oil respectively. It took roughly six months, but Jamie became "a different child" according to his mother. His balance and motor problems improved along with his behavioral problems.

Where Are the Children Going?

Today, we better understand the importance of childhood in forming a complex and superbly functioning brain. Yet it is during this vital period of brain formation that the current dietary habits of children are most suspect. There is increasing evidence that today's youth get far too much saturated fat and far too little of the unsaturated fatty acids needed to nurture the brain to its greatest potential.

Scientists writing in *Nutrition Reviews* found the following with respect to eating habits of U.S. kids:[21]

- An overwhelming majority exceed the recommended thirty percent of their calories from fat.
- Most obtained more than ten percent of their calories from *saturated* fat, which is excessive.
- The major sources of fat were meat and dairy products—devoid of essential fatty acids, especially neural fatty acids.
- Substantial calories came from desserts, candy, snacks, and chips—high in trans fatty acids.

These trends in childhood consumption mirror our adult habits. Parents must take responsibility for their idividual personal eating habits if they wish to bring their children's eating habits to a point of balancing fats and oils in healthy ways. School systems that provide lunch must also be aware of the crucial need for fatty acid balance in brain development.

TEENAGERS: MAKING THE YEARS FLOW SMOOTHLY

During adolescence, the brain continues to change, forming new connections and expanding its myelination. However, the brain's plasticity, or ability to change, is not as it was in early childhood. By age eighteen, the brain's plasticity has declined, but the power of its connections has increased. Essential fatty acids appear necessary to nurture this ongoing evolution of the adolescent's brain.

Unfortunately, the trend among many adolescents is toward high-saturated-fat food that is rich in trans fatty acids. On the other side of this coin are children who restrict their diets in various ways for personal reasons. Young athletes are a good example. Gymnasts restrict calories to remain petite and "fit." Wrestlers restrict calories to remain within their weight class. Runners load up on carbohydrates and restrict fat (including fatty acids) with the mistaken belief that this improves endurance. Football players and bodybuilders load up on foods high in protein and saturated fat, consuming very low amounts of unsaturated fatty acids. As we'll see below, such personal choices may come with a price.

Starving the Body, Starving the Mind: Dangerous Choices for Young Girls

Popular culture has placed such high expectations on young girls to be thin and look glamorous that is it almost impossible to achieve peak nutrition. Images of thin, curvaceous women drive young girls to strive, through starvation, for the "sexy" look seen on magazine covers throughout the world. Is it any wonder that, according to one study, sixty percent of girls aged six to twelve develop distorted body image and overestimate their body weight.[22] Such distorted self-image leads young girls who are not overweight to needlessly pursue restrictive diets. One report on 500 ten-year-old girls revealed that a startling eighty-one percent were (or already had been) on a diet of some kind.[23]

The obsession with being thin has led to a revolt against fat in all its forms. Diets that result from such attitudes are notoriously low in fat, especially omega-3 fatty acids. In essence, the young girls driven to thinness by the glamour culture may be starving themselves of essential fatty acids.

I recently consulted with such a girl. She was a bright seventeen-year-old given to bouts of aggression, moodiness, panic, and uncontrollable weeping. She suffered from severe chronic tiredness. These symptoms were no surprise considering her dietary habits. Her mother remarked, "Tania is so afraid of fat that she often eats little more than a handful of 'fat-free' soda crackers."

The brain of a young girl is still developing and maturing. By starving herself of calories, she likely restricts fatty acids that the brain needs to continue weaving its complex web of neurons. If young girls restrict their fatty acid intake during this critical time, they may compromise brain maturation and set a dangerous pattern for the future. In later chapters, we will explore how fatty acid imbalance may contribute to aggression, violence, mood disorders, and behavior changes. A curious question arises regarding whether dangerous "fatty-acid-deficient" diets of adolescence contribute to some of the huge difficulties faced by teenagers today? Might some of the social upheaval observed in today's teen culture be due to fundamental changes in brain structure brought about by years of marginal intake of the brain's main structural fats?

The second part of this matter concerns future generations. As previously discussed, some scientists believe that adolescence is perhaps the most important time for young girls to develop the peak nutrient reserves that will one day nourish a child during pregnancy. If a young girl robs herself of neural fatty acids as she matures, she may not have adequate reserves to foster peak brain development in her offspring when she eventually bears a child.

Taken a step further, it is important to recall that many adolescents who live on low EFA diets may have received inadequate fatty acids as infants and small children as well. Because of this, they can ill afford to sustain a poor intake of essential fatty acids during another critical phase of their brain development.

Alcohol and Brain-Fats in the Teenage Years

Adolescence is also a time when children begin to experiment with alcohol. It is important to remember the work of Drs. Pawlosky and Salem at the National Institutes of Health. They have studied the effects of alcohol on the nervous system and note that alcohol may disrupt the fatty acids (especially DHA) of brain membranes. They write, "Studies of lower concentrations of DHA (22:6n3) in the nervous system is associated with a loss of nervous system function."[24] According to neurologist Jean-Marie Bourre, the effect of alcohol on the brain in someone who is already low in fatty acids like alpha-linolenic acid (one can also include DHA) is even more pronounced.

ADULTS: MAINTAINING PEAK BRAIN PERFORMANCE

All of the critical periods leading up to adulthood are important to forming the healthy foundation upon which adulthood will be built. The time of youth has an enormous impact on the body's health and on organ reserve. The passage of time also means that the stress of life that is so much a part of modern existence may influence our current state of health. Adulthood is a critical period because many of our rebuilding and repairing processes are not as efficient as in the peak of our youth.

As we age, the ability to manufacture long-chain neural fatty acids becomes less efficient because the enzymes needed to convert them begin to wear out. This means that dietary sources become more important. As we age, the cumulative effects of free radicals on brain tissue becomes more evident. With increasing free radical activity comes increasing lipid peroxidation, or rancid fats. Replacing damaged fatty acids in brain membranes may be important in retaining brain function as we get older. It is adulthood when many of the brain changes that began in our youth begin to show themselves.

The importance of fatty acid balance has recently been highlighted by the observations of a group of scientists working independently on the role of DHA on mental function in adulthood.

Dr. David Kyle has reviewed data from the Framingham study and has preliminary evidence that those with low DHA in adulthood were more likely to develop dementia as they age.[25] Dr. Peter Marksubury, of the University of Kentucky, has unpublished observations that Alzheimer's patients have thirty percent lower DHA in their brains.[26] Dr. Paavo Rickkinen noted that aged rats have lower brain DHA, which corresponded with a poorer EEG (electroencephalogram) response.[27] Dr. Ernst Schaefer, of the Human Nutrition Center on Aging at Tufts University, has discovered that a low level of DHA is a significant risk factor for dementia.[28]

These and other observations point to DHA and other fatty acids as critical nutrients in the adult years. In the following chapters, we will explore the dynamic effect of fatty acids on the brain's performance and the strategies one can use to keep brain function at its peak.

PART III

HOW FATS AND OILS INFLUENCE THE BRAIN'S PERFORMANCE

In this section, I explore the specific aspects of the brain's function that are affected by fats and oils. As you review this section you'll read some profound stories. While the stories and the research are very exciting and may compel you to experiment freely with fatty acids, there are several words of caution I would like you to consider.

CAUTIONS

1. Though I may describe cases in which a specific fatty acid brought about a desired outcome, another person with similar symptoms may require a somewhat different balance of fats. For example, DHA may help an adult with mood or behavior problems, but another may require GLA. One child with attention problems may respond to flax oil, while another may get worse on flax oil, but respond to primrose oil.

In some disorders of the brain, long-chain fatty acids such as DHA actually accumulate in high levels. Children with autism, for example, often respond poorly when given long-chain fatty acids or phosphatidylserine, even though they may appear to need them. A similar situation sometimes arises with seizures where long-chain fatty acids worsen the condition.

Laboratory tests are sometimes needed to determine the specific fatty acids needed in a given circumstance. Anyone with an existing condition of the brain is advised to seek the advice of a health care professional who is knowledgeable in this area. Appendix C contains a referral number for clinicians who are generally knowledgeable in nutrition.

2. If you take fatty acid supplements and experience any problems whatsoever, discontinue the supplement and consult a health professional *knowledgeable in fatty acid nutrition*. While fatty acids are generally *very* safe to work with, someone with an existing brain disorder may be extremely sensitive to the molecular form of fatty acid being used. This will make more sense if you refer back to Chapters Three and Four for a discussion of the different fatty acid pathways.

3. Taking supplemental fatty acids is only part of the puzzle of restoring brain fatty acid balance; making sure the enzymes and transport systems work properly is vital. In addition, certain trace minerals, vitamins, and accessory nutrients must be used to make the system fully functional. Avoiding harmful fats is also important. Sometimes, specific saturated fats are needed.

4. Understand that while we know a great deal more than we did only five years ago about fatty acids and the brain, we are still in the early stages. Therefore, the level of sophistication presented in the following chapters can be expected to improve with each passing year. In addition, many of the most learned people in the field of fatty acids and brain chemistry disagree about the significance of certain findings. Thus, you may wish to pursue these alternative viewpoints as well.

5. Fatty acids are extremely potent biological substances. The ratios in which we consume them are very important. You can just as easily create imbalance by consuming too much of a given fatty acid. The key is to know what you are doing and make intelligent decisions.

6. The distinction I draw between mental and physical illness, or between neurodegenerative and behavioral disorders is somewhat artificial. I believe that these distinctions are not as well-defined as we like to believe, but that we use them for ease of understanding or communicating our ideas.

7. Nutrition is only one part of the equation. There are many non-nutritional factors that merge to influence brain function.

8. Fatty acids can change the dosage requirements for drugs. This has been shown, for example, with antidepressants such as Prozac and with insulin. There may be such affects with many drugs, perhaps, because of the way the right fatty acids can improve the linking of receptors with neurotransmitters and other substances. Fatty acids should also be used with great caution by those on anticoagulant (blood thinning) drugs. If you are on medication, you should speak with your doctor about monitoring your drug dose and fatty acid needs.

9. Fatty acid uptake into the nervous system can be very slow. Though some of the patients described in this book recovered very quickly from their ailments, others may take much longer. It is not unusual for improvement to take six months to two years

10. Additional vitamin E and other antioxidants must always be used whenever fatty acid supplements are used. This helps protect against the formation of rancid fats (peroxidized lipids) in the body.

11. While unsaturated fatty acids have been emphasized, therapy with *specific* saturated fats, is sometimes needed.

CHAPTER 9

PROTECTING MOOD AND BEHAVIOR

Henrietta had been through all of this before. As the fall months approached, her mood began to sink. It became increasingly difficult for her to conduct her work as a mental health counselor. With each passing day, the urge to simply lie down and escape the world was stronger than the previous day. Henrietta had passing suicidal urges, which she fought by retreating into sleep. Her depression was severe and required medication. Yet, she was not prepared to consider the medication as a long-term solution.

Henrietta turned to nutritionist Robert Crayhon in New York. A nutritional strategy was designed, which initially had modest impact. In an attempt to more carefully tailor her program, she began taking supplemental doses of the fats EPA, DHA, and phosphatidylserine. The effect on her mood was powerful. As a mental health counselor she knew all too well the signs, symptoms, and drudgery of a mood disorder. A sufferer herself, she was acutely sensitive to anything that might bring about change to the downward spiral. Essential fatty acids became the cornerstone of her recovery.[1]

This is not unlike the experience of young Colin, a nine-year-old given to bouts of aggression. He grew up in a family that raised him in a gentle, non-violent manner. There was no television or video games in the home and none of the things that provide images of violence and aggression. Yet, Colin was unreasonably aggressive with his siblings, classmates, and others.

His parents, one of whom was a physician, provided a diet that was well-balanced and free of junk food. Even this did not seem to curb Colin's aggression.

Colin's diet was modified to improve the intake of omega-3 fatty acids. In addition, he began taking DHA and GLA supplements daily. Since beginning the fatty acid protocol, the change in his aggression has been inspiring. As his mother describes him, "He is calm, courteous, and considerate. We experience very little in the way of aggressive outbursts."

The experiences of Colin and Henrietta add to a growing body of evidence linking essential fatty acids to brain function. The relationship is being clarified by discoveries in the emerging field of what some refer to as nutritional neuroscience.

Further defining this field in 1995, two scientists from the National Institutes of Health published a landmark paper entitled "Dietary Polyunsaturated Fatty Acids and Depression." In their review of many scientific papers on the subject, Drs. Joseph Hibbeln and Norman Salem write, "We postulate that adequate long chain polyunsaturated fatty acids, particularly DHA, may reduce the rate of depression just as omega-3 polyunsaturated fatty acids may reduce coronary artery disease."

In their treatise they go beyond depression, suggesting that a host of mood and behavioral disorders may be affected by dietary fatty acids. They state, "Although we present a case for the association between depression and DHA deficiency, the relations between dietary polyunsaturated fatty acids, affective and psychotic disorders, as well as type A personality traits, impulsivity, and violence, may also be important."[2]

Hibbeln and Salem are not the first to propose such a link. In the early 1980s, Donald Rudin, M.D., published some of the most intriguing and provocative work linking fatty acid imbalance to a number of psychological conditions. David Horrobin, M.D., of Nova Scotia, has produced similarly noteworthy work on the subject of fatty acids and brain disorders.

The findings and conclusions of these and other researchers have set the tone for a new and provocative undertaking. They may shed a common light on the origins of a vast array of conditions that, up until now, have been viewed as separate and distinct entities.

Certainly, there are many factors that come to bear on our mood and emotions. Life circumstances, belief systems, patterns of our upbringing, relationships with family members—these all profoundly influence our emotional state. Yet, the potentially powerful effect of fatty acids opens an entirely new window of opportunity.

One such condition is depression, a malady whose incidence has increased in every generation since 1900.[3] What is it that compels us to believe depression may be related to dietary fat and essential fatty acids?

IS DEPRESSION DUE TO FATTY ACID IMBALANCE?

Not long ago, I was in Philadelphia presenting a lecture at the Institutes for the Achievement of Human Potential world symposium. This is a group that has helped shatter some of the old myths about the limits of our brain capacity. Gathered was an assembly of neurosurgeons, space medicine specialists, therapists, nutritionists, biochemists, and educators. My topic was entitled "Essential Fatty Acids, Neural Architecture, and Nervous System Disease." My greatest challenge was to compress the volumes of material and still capture the essence of this fascinating story in a mere ninety-minute talk.

When the question and answer period finally arrived, a physician from China rose from her seat to remind me that, for centuries in her country, fish has been considered an important food to eat for a "balanced, happy mood and better mental performance." She was correct, of course.

Observing cultural practices has always given us keen insight into solutions to our problems. A curious clue linking brain-fats to depression came from cultures consuming large amounts of fish— they had lower rates of depression.[4] North American and European peoples had rates of depression nearly tenfold higher than the people of Taiwan, a fish-consuming society.[5]

The rate of major depression was nearly seven times higher in North America (depending upon the city chosen) than in Hong Kong.[6] In one Japanese study, the rate of depression was below one percent.[7] In a rural fishing village in Japan, psychiatrists could find no one with major depression.[8]

Years ago, we may have had no possible way to explain why fish consumption might affect mood. However, when we consider that fish are the richest source of neural fatty acids such as DHA and that these fatty acids may influence the function of nerve transmission, it begins to make sense. Beyond the cultural evidence, there are additional clues.

An Ancient Recipe for Depression?

A curious book was published in 1652 entitled *The Anatomy of Melancholy*. Melancholy, of course, is an old term used to describe a condition similar to what we would today call depression. In this book, the author recommends a low-fat diet, borage oil, and consumption of fish. For severe cases, he advocated consuming cow brains.[9]

Borage oil, fish, and cow brains? This seemingly odd combination might be enough to send anyone running for the mouthwash and antacids. But, on closer inspection, and based on what we are beginning to understand about brain-fats, it becomes more plausible.

Fish, of course, has DHA. Borage oil is very high in GLA (gamma-linolenic acid), not a neural fat, but does have a role in regulating eicosanoids that affect the brain. Cow brains* would be very high in DHA, arachidonic acid, phosphatidylcholine (PC), and phosphatidylserine (PS). Together, these substances just might have a positive influence on depression. Biochemically, it makes sense. Neurologically, it makes sense.

---

*Interestingly, many cultures have advocated consuming animal brains to improve mental function, balance mood, and heal problems of the "nerves." However, I'm not advocating cow brains as a therapeutic solution. I only use it here as a historical reference.

Depression and Fats out of Balance

In Chapter Four, we learned about the importance of maintaining a *balance* of omega-6 to omega-3 fatty acids. As this balance shifts in one direction or another there is great tendency toward development of disease. In most modern cultures, the balance has shifted in one direction: high n-6 to n-3 ratio. In other words, too much omega-6, too little omega-3.

When Dr. Peter Adams and his group in Melbourne, Australia studied people with moderate to severe depression, they discovered a trend that we are beginning to see all too often. The omega-6 to omega-3 ratio was elevated and this correlated with symptoms of depression. Dr. Adam's group concluded their assessment by suggesting nutritional supplementation may have benefit in depressed people by balancing the n-6 to n-3 ratio.[10]

Belgian physician Michael Maes also found that people with depression had significantly higher n-6 to n-3 fatty acid ratios in their blood and suggested that, "A supplementation trial of fish oil in major depression is warranted."[11]

The Case of Janet

Janet was a fifty-three-year-old woman who suffered from severe depression. She had been on a number of prescription drugs over the years, some of which gave her relief. However, she was uncomfortable with the thought of relying on drugs for the rest of her life and sought alternatives in the realm of nutrition. Laboratory analysis of her blood plasma and red blood cell fatty acids showed a number of abnormalities, which included low EPA, low DHA, low ALA (alpha-linolenic acid), and an elevated ratio of omega-6 to omega-3 fatty acids.

Therapy was based on restoring balance to the fatty acids and their pathways. This involved cofactor nutrients such as zinc, magnesium, niacin, and vitamin C, as well as essential fatty acids of the omega-3 variety. Dietary changes were also recommended: restricting meat and consuming cold-water fish such as salmon.

Over a period of months, her symptoms began to improve substantially. Though she still required some medication, she needed it much less than previously. This is a pattern seen in some studies. Essential fatty acids seem to augment the action of some antidepressant drugs.

Blood Sludge and Depression

Factors that cause the blood to thicken can slow oxygen to the brain and also affect mood. Charles Glueck, M.D., medical director of the Cholesterol Center of Jewish Hospital in Cincinnati asserts that elevated blood cholesterol and triglycerides are strongly correlated with the incidence of what are called affective disorders. This includes depression, manic depression, schizoaffective disorder, and others. Elevated triglycerides are also associated with hostility and aggression. It holds true for adults and children.

Glueck states that "We have shown that in patients with high triglycerides who were in a depressive state, the more you lower the triglycerides, the more you alleviate the depression."[12] He bases his assertions on an important study he and his colleagues conducted prior to 1994. They found that thirty-nine percent of his study group with familial hypertriglyceridemia had mild-to-severe depression. While on a low-fat diet (ten to fifteen percent fat) ninety-one percent were rated normal with regard to depression.[13]

This was a circumstance in which a low-fat diet was helpful. We should always keep in mind, however, that low-fat diets that also restrict essential fatty acids can be a problem for many people. Ensuring proper intake of omega-3 fatty acids can also help reduce triglycerides and prevent blood sludging.[14]

The Story of Terry

Terry is living testament to the ideas of Dr. Glueck. Terry was an accountant in his mid-forties who had become fidgety, anxious, depressed, and irritable. He was inclined toward quick-tempered outbursts and was intolerant of his children. This, not surprisingly, concerned his wife a great deal. What concerned Terry, however, was his deteriorating memory, lack of interest, and sleep difficulties. It all began to affect his work.

Blood tests revealed sharply elevated triglycerides and choles-terol. In his dietary analysis he consumed mostly junk food: cook-ies, doughnuts, candy bars, french fries, chips, soda pop, and take-out fried chicken. It was full of saturated fat and contained no food sources of omega-3 fatty acids.

By making dietary changes to reduce saturated fat, eliminate trans fatty acids, and increase omega-3 fatty acids his life slowly began to return to normal. As his blood-fats came down and his brain-fat intake went up, his mood returned to a more balanced state.

Postpartum Depression: Is There A Fatty Acid Link?

Postpartum depression affects a large number of women following childbirth. Though no one knows why, the risk seems to increase with each successive pregnancy. Given what we're learning about fatty acids and mood disorders, one wonders about postpartum depression. Adding further intrigue to the question is the findings of fatty acid abnormality following pregnancy. Recall the studies of Dr. Monique Al and her colleagues who found that DHA stores declined during pregnancy and that blood levels of DHA became lower were each successive child.[15] Drs. Joseph Hibbeln and Nor-man Salem also commented on the subject of declining fatty acids in pregnancy. They wrote, "This relative maternal depletion of DHA may be one of the complex factors leading to increased risk of depression in women of childbearing age and in postpartum periods."[16]

I have listened to the lament of many women who've said, "I have never been the same since my last child." Given our new knowledge of fatty acids, this lament should be met with an inves-tigation of fatty acid status. A trial of omega-3 fatty acids may be in order.

Obsessive-Compulsive Disorder

There also appears to be a relationship between obsessive-compul-sive disorder (OCD) and pregnancy. Dr. Fugen Neziroglu and col-leagues noted that during interviews and treatment of over 500 patients with obsessive-compulsive disorder it was observed that "the onset for many women appeared to be during pregnancy."

They reported on another group of women with OCD in which sixty-nine percent reported their OCD either began with or was worsened by some aspect of their pregnancy, birth, or care of their children. In yet another group, thirty-nine percent were found to have developed their first symptoms of OCD during or after their pregnancy.[17]

Men, children, and women who have never had children also develop OCD, so the solution to this problem may not be so simple. Yet, if there is a link between obsessive-compulsive disorder and pregnancy, might it be due to the same fatty acid decline purported to occur in postpartum depression? There is not much reseach exploring this link. However, in one case of a woman in her mid-thirties with OCD, blood levels of fatty acids were abnormal. Medication and psychotherapy has helped her gradually improve, but addition of the brain-fats phosphatidylserine and DHA to her treatment has made an enormous difference.

Depression in Multiple Sclerosis

People with multiple sclerosis (MS) are particularly prone to depression. This is not unexpected when you consider the difficulty of living with such a disabling illness. Yet, people with MS seem to suffer from depression at a much higher rate than people with other illnesses with similar degrees of disability.[18]

When scientists studied the brains of people with MS, they found a marked reduction in brain-fats such as DHA. They also found low levels of omega-3 fatty acids in blood and almost no omega-3 fatty acids stored in fat tissues.[19] Findings like these have prompted several studies in which omega-3 fatty acids are given to people with MS. These studies have often shown that mood and perception of quality of life improve. Taken together, it provides further evidence suggesting a link between essential fatty acids and neuropsychological illness.[20]

PS in Depression and the Winter Blues

You may recall our discussion of phosphatidylserine (PS) from Chapter Four. It is one of the structural units of nerve-cell membranes and is increasingly being used as a nutritional supplement in problems of the brain. Contained within the structure of PS are essential fatty acids. In one study of people with unipolar depression, blood levels of PS were below normal.[21] Supplementation with PS has given people relief from depressive symptoms.[22]

Seasonal affective disorder, the "winter blues," generally occurs in Northern climates where winter daylight exposure is short. Evidence is building that brain-fats can be helpful in this condition as well. When phosphatidylserine was given to elderly people with the "winter blues," they experienced significant improvement in their moods. In addition, they had improvement in memory and ability to manipulate information.[23] This study is consistent with others that have shown improvement in seasonal depression with PS supplementation.[24]

FEAR AND PHOBIA: WHEN RAY RETURNED TO LIFE

Ray was a successful musician who had spent many years in the public eye, an arena in which he had become quite comfortable. However, very slowly he began to develop fears that so paralyzed him that he could no longer perform in public. As his struggles progressed he became increasingly afraid to leave his home for any purpose. By 1996, his fears had so overwhelmed him that he was unable to leave his home or engage in any of the activities of his normal life. He had become a prisoner of his fear, a fate of those who suffer from agoraphobia.

During this period of declining health, Ray also suffered from psoriasis. Psoriasis is a skin condition that is very difficult to treat, but has been associated with essential fatty acid imbalance. Some cases improve with fatty acid supplementation.

Ray began taking the fatty acid DHA at a dose of 200 mg per day. Over a period of just two short months his fears began to subside. Most gratifying was that his fear of going outdoors or out in public vanished. He had come so far in his recovery that he scheduled a trip to Branson, Missouri, a mecca for country music enthusiasts.

An interesting lesson arises from Ray's experience. Many people with altered mood and behavior, if one looks closely enough, also have skin, hair, or nail changes that hint at fatty acid insufficiency. We should always be aware of these hidden clues. Further, while this is only one case, it is part of an expanding web of clinical experience that reveals how fatty acid imbalance can affect our most fundamental emotions. Ray is only one among many individuals whose phobias have responded to fatty acid supplementation.

TIRED ALL THE TIME: EFA AND CHRONIC FATIGUE

Chronic fatigue is often accompanied by a sea of emotional changes. In 1990, researchers from Scotland and Canada reported on their study of essential fatty acid supplementation in fatigued patients with exhaustion, weakness, and poor concentration. In the fatigued patients, red cell levels of omega-3 and omega-6 fatty acids were well below normal. Each was then given a supplement containing GLA, EPA, and DHA. Fatty acid supplementation caused improvement in eighty-five percent after three months. Not only did symptoms improve, but red cell fatty acid levels returned to normal.[25] In contrast, improvement occurred in only seventeen percent of the placebo group.

ATTENTION PROBLEMS AND HYPERACTIVITY

An estimated fifteen million people in the U.S. suffer from symptoms of distractibility, impulsivity, and excess nervous energy. For them, life can be a difficult and constant struggle. In some classrooms in the United States, over one-half the children are on the stimulant drug Ritalin. We tend to think of hyperactivity and attention deficit in terms of children, but these problems affect adults as well. One must ask, "What are the underlying factors that give rise to this condition?" Additionally, "What are the consequences to our evolving culture should we not find a solution?"

Signs of Imbalance

For years doctors have observed the general signs of fatty acid imbalance in people with hyperactive symptoms: dry skin, increased thirst, frequent urination, dry unmanageable hair, and allergies. Then, in 1987, doctors had some evidence of abnormal brain-fats. Dr. E. A. Mitchell and colleagues found that children with attention deficit and hyperactivity had low blood levels of DHA and arachidonic acid, two of the key brain-fats.[26]

Further evidence surfaced at Purdue University in 1995 when researchers found low levels of DHA and arachidonic acid. In addition, children with ADHD (attention deficit hyperactivity disorder) were found to have a higher omega-6 to omega-3 ratio. Remember that when the omega-6 to omega-3 ratio gets too high it may lead to lower available brain-fats. It appears to set the stage for improper balance of long-chain fatty acids in the nervous system.[27] This is reminiscent of the depressed adults studied by Drs. Adams and Maes who had a high n-6 to n-3 ratio.

In the Purdue study, children who had been breast-fed were less likely to have ADHD. Further, the longer the period of breast-feeding, the lower the likelihood of having ADHD. Remember that breast milk is high in fatty acids such as GLA, ALA, DHA, and arachidonic acid, but most formula, up to 1997, contained none of these fatty acids.

Then, in 1996, the Purdue group published their study on ninety-six boys, looking for a relationship between omega-3 fatty acids and behavior. Those with lower omega-3 fatty acids in their blood were found to have more learning and behavior problems than those whose levels were normal. The most common behavioral difficulties in those with low omega-3 fatty acids included temper tantrums, impulsivity, anxiety, hyperactivity, and conduct.[28]

In the studies above, there was a common finding of several fatty acid insufficiency signs. Most common signs included excessive thirst, frequent urination, dry hair, and dry skin. In fact, according to Dr. J. Burgess, of Purdue, children with these signs *and* the symptoms of ADHD were most likely to have abnormal fatty acid profiles.

Sidney Baker, M.D. is a former professor at Yale University School of Medicine and is a leader in the field of nutritional and environmental medicine. In my many conversations with Dr. Baker I have known him to be a constant source of wisdom, common sense, and medical knowledge. He has worked with many people who suffer from attention problems and hyperactivity, and believes fatty acid balance is among the most crucial issues. His advice: always look for changes in the skin. It is often the signpost that points to fatty acid imbalance.

A Lesson for Adults

Attention deficit and hyperactivity disorder continue to affect many people as they reach adulthood. In fact, mood disorders in adulthood appear to be more common if hyperactivity or attention deficit existed in childhood. Might essential fatty acids have been at the core of the problem? As an adult, might there be refuge in improving the intake of essential fatty acids? In my opinion, both children and adults with learning, mood, attention, and hyperactivity problems can benefit from balancing their fatty acid intake. Certain key supplements, which we'll discuss later, may also be of great help.

VIOLENCE AND AGGRESSION

Scientists learned long ago that fatty acid imbalance may be associated with violence and aggression. Studies showed that low-fat, low-cholesterol diets led to:

- More violent, aggressive behavior.[30]
- Changes in brain neurotransmitter function (serotonin).[31]
- More violent, aggressive behavior, and less social interaction. Reduced serotonin action in the brain.[32]

These findings, in some ways, mirror what is happening in our society. The most startling results, however, are revealed in a study of Capuchin monkeys who were raised on a diet using corn oil as the sole source of fatty acids. Behavior in the group degenerated so badly that, by age two, some of the animals demonstrated self-mutilation behavior.[33]

This omega-3 deficient diet was thought to be acceptably balanced in fat at the time of the study. Yet, there was no doubt about its negative effects on the brain. Curiously, corn oil was the principal source of unsaturated fatty acids in our own culture for many years.

It seems that low-fat diets like the ones described above caused changes in brain chemistry because they did not address the brain's need for *essential fatty acids*, especially omega-3 fatty acids. These low-fat diets apparently led to changes in the brain that manifested as increased violent and aggressive behavior. We will see later how DHA supplementation may reduce aggression in healthy adults.

When doctors studied violent offenders in a prison system they found fatty acid abnormalities were common. Blood measurements revealed very low DHA in violent, antisocial men. Another common finding: serum cholesterol was very low. All consumed alcohol.[34] We know from previous chapters that alcohol:

- Damages fatty acids (DHA) in brain membranes.
- Blocks the enzymes that enable one to form our own brain fats such as DHA from the parent dietary fatty acids such as linolenic acid.
- Blocks the enzymes needed to make the messenger PGE1.

Recall the comments of Dr. R. J. Pawlosky, who has studied the brain effects of alcohol. He notes that alcohol may disrupt the fatty membrane of nerve cells, reducing their content of the critical brain fat DHA. He further states that "lower concentration of DHA in the nervous system is associated with a loss of nervous system function. Alcoholics are prone to many cognitive disorders involving loss of memory, inability to concentrate, and dementia. Some of these functions may be modulated, in part, by DHA concentrations. The alcohol-induced loss of neural DHA may provide a mechanism underlying aspects of this neurological impairment."[35]

SCHIZOPHRENIA AND THE FAT CONNECTION

Schizophrenia may also involve fatty acid imbalance. The World Health Organization coordinated a study showing that schizophrenia was more severe in countries whose total fat consumption was very high and less severe in nations whose fat consumption was low. High animal fat intake usually correlates with low intake of long-chain unsaturated fatty acids, especially omega-3 fatty acids like DHA, the ones required for brain architecture and proper brain function.

The researchers concluded that dietary fat intake appeared not to influence *whether* one developed schizophrenia, but it strongly influenced the severity of schizophrenia.[36] This may suggest that schizophrenia has a strong genetic component that is greatly influenced by the type of fat made available to the nervous system via the diet.

Schizophrenia and Fatty-Acid Supplements

Schizophrenia is often divided into subgroups: one with so-called negative- and one with so-called positive signs. Negative signs include apathy and withdrawal, while positive signs include thought disorder, hallucinations, or delusions. In a study published in *Schizophrenia Research*, people with "negative" signs had much lower omega-3 fatty acids such as DHA in their blood. Those with "positive" signs showed no such differences.[37]

Several studies have been conducted to determine whether omega-3 fatty acid supplementation improved the course of schizophrenia. In one study, when psychiatrists gave ten grams of fish oil for six weeks to people with schizophrenia there was an improvement in twenty different schizophrenic symptoms. In addition, the blood levels of n-3 fatty acids improved.[38,39]

GLA, from evening primrose oil, has also been used with some success in schizophrenia.[40]

THE STRESS RESPONSE

Some doctors have argued that the only time critical brain-fats such as DHA are needed is during pregnancy, infancy, and child-hood—times when the brain is forming. However, we've seen in this chapter that people with certain mood disorders have low brain fats and that some people with mood disorders benefit from brain-fat supplementation. In previous chapters, we saw that many sources of free radicals may damage the brain's fatty acids and that trans fatty acids can be taken up into the brain. More-over, we need only look at the stress research and see that there are many life circumstances that might lead to alteration of fatty acids in the brain. This probably makes lifetime, regular consumption of brain-fats very important to long-term health and vitality.

Numerous studies have shown that stress of various forms causes damage to the delicate fatty acids of the brain.[41,42,43] The hormones secreted as part of the stress response are well known to disrupt the use and formation of the brain's fatty acids. Brain changes due to stress resemble the effects of aging on the brain and can even cause shrinking of the cerebral cortex. In short, chronic stress causes premature aging of the brain.[44]

Fatty Acid Supplements and Stress

Fatty acid supplements may be helpful tools in blunting the stress response or in restoring brain-fats following stressful periods. When you're under stress, your body reacts in certain predictable ways that can be measured. Changes in blood pressure, heart rate, and skin temperature are among these changes. When individuals were supplemented with borage oil and fish oil, sources of GLA and DHA respectively, it reversed the rise in blood pressure often associated with psychological stress.[45] In two other studies, doc-tors found that PS supplementation significantly reduced the stress hormone response to physical stress.[46,47]

Conclusions About Stress and Brain Fats

While we have more questions than answers, it seems clear that stress has an adverse effect on the brain over the long term. Some of this is probably brought about by changes in the fatty acids. Hibbeln and Salem of the National Institutes of Health have addressed this issue in their very important work and suggest that stress may contribute to the following:[48]

- Destruction (rancidity) of long-chain essential fatty acids in the brain.
- Inadequate replacement of these lost fatty acids with appropriate fatty acids.
- Eventual depletion of nervous system long-chain fatty acids, which may lead to behavioral disorders such as depression.

If their assessment is accurate, it may give us a powerful new tool in management of stress-related disorders. It may also call for supplementation with key fatty acid products to treat a wide range of conditions related to stress.

Beyond this, it may suggest that even though fatty acid levels in youth may be necessary to protect the brain later in life, events throughout life may require that key neural fatty acids be regularly or periodically replaced through diet or supplementation. In cases where neural fatty acids have not been provided in youth, effects of stress may be more pronounced and the need for supplementation may be even more important.

HOPE FOR BALANCING MOOD AND BEHAVIOR

We are only in the early stages of discovering how important essential fatty acids are to brain structure and function. This new knowledge holds great promise for the future of individuals and perhaps even society.

CHAPTER 10

PROTECTING THE BRAIN AGAINST NEUROLOGICAL DISEASES

Daniel was a forty-five-year-old electrician from Minnesota. In 1993, he began to notice weakness and trembling in his right hand whenever he reached to gesture or pick up an object. This progressed to gradual paralysis of the right arm, right leg, and face. By 1996, he was unable to tie his shoe or button his shirt. The fine movements of his hand began to give way to rigidity, which made it difficult to do the most basic things like writing with a pencil. Disturbing numbness and tingling of his arm and hand was a constant reminder of something gone awry.

His neurologists performed an MRI (magnetic resonance imaging scan of the brain) and found that a portion of brain called the pons-midbrain junction was being damaged. Structures in this area are critical to controlling movement. The prognosis was very bad. Daniel's neurologists told him to expect gradual worsening and cautioned him against expectations of any improvement. The cause was unknown and there was no effective treatment.

In 1996, he entered the office of Dr. Virginia Shapiro of Duluth, Minnesota. She had recently begun working with some of her more difficult neurological cases using specific essential fatty acids. Dr. Shapiro determined that Daniel was a good candidate for fatty-acid therapy and placed him on the fatty acid DHA at a dose of 300 mg per day. His initial gradual improvement was encouraging. He slowly regained better control over his limbs. As the tremors improved, he gradually regained his ability to write, button his clothing, and conduct other fine movements. Over a six-month period, there was striking improvement. As of this writing he is able to do everything for himself and continues to improve—this all in a man who was expected to degenerate indefinitely.[1]

Another case further underscores the excitement that is being generated by our new knowledge about fatty acids, the brain, and the nervous system. Sean suffered from severe seizures and a condition called global developmental delay that left him partially paralyzed and frequently unable to interact within his world. He appeared normal until about eight months of age. Then, for unknown reasons, his health began to deteriorate. On the day of his first visit, this now-six-year-old boy had to be carried into the office. Sean's mother reported that he rarely walked at home under his own initiative and only after great prompting did he walk at all. His muscle tone was so poor that he was unable to sit on the examining table under his own power. Even at age six, Sean rarely slept through the night. Intractable seizures made Sean's life a constant struggle and his condition dominated his family's life.

Sean had received various forms of drug treatment for his seizures with modest success, but there was little being done to impact his developmental and motor problems. Here is where fatty acids became important. Sean was placed on a DHA supplement at a dose of about 150 to 200 mg per day. After the first day of therapy, he slept through the night. This was no proof of anything, but an encouraging sign nonetheless. Over the course of the next month, however, his improvement was unexpectedly good for someone with such a severe disorder. Within four weeks of DHA therapy, rather than being carried, he walked into the clinic under his own power. Sean was able to sit up on the examination table without being held by his mother. More encouraging yet, at home he was walking under his own initiative and did not require the kind of prodding once routine.[2]

The improvement in Sean's hypotonia and in other specific areas has been exciting. His seizures, however, have not improved. Time will tell whether fatty acids have an eventual impact on this aspect of his nervous system. Yet, his story illustrates two important points. First, nervous system problems can be enormously complex. Sometimes, balancing brain-fats is only part of the equation. Second, it illustrates how profoundly the nervous system *can* be changed when nervous system fatty-acid insufficiency is corrected by supplementation.

Daniel and Sean experienced problems with their sensory and motor systems. Our sensory system consists of smell, sight, taste, touch, hearing, pain, pressure sense, and others ways of interpreting the world around us. Our motor system is responsible for control of our muscles and tendons. Ability to move through our world is determined by the motor system. Integration of our sensory and motor systems is what allows us to flow harmoniously through our environment and live in a world of such complex surroundings.

In the cases of Daniel and young Sean, DHA supplementation had a dramatic and pronounced effect on their abilities to sense and to move. In a relatively short period of time, DHA appeared to change the function of the sensory and motor parts of their brains. We cannot say for certain exactly how DHA was able to do this. But from what we know of the brain's structure and with what we've learned from scientific studies over the past twenty years, we can speculate that proper fatty-acid balance was restored to the very delicate membranes of the nerve fibers themselves. By restoring balance, the neurons may have begun firing more normally, which yielded better control of muscles and other functions.

In the above examples, DHA was the nutrient that improved brain function. However, in other circumstances, it could have been GLA (gamma-linolenic acid), ALA (alpha-linolenic acid), or a combination of fatty substances. Careful consideration must be given to the existing fatty-acid balance in people with such disorders before simply beginning supplementation. The reason for this will become more clear as you read further in this chapter.

I predict that as we learn more about the role of fats and oils in the brain that this knowledge will fundamentally change how we look at disorders of the nervous system. One such brain disease is multiple sclerosis.

MULTIPLE SCLEROSIS

Because seventy-five percent of the myelin sheath covering nerves is fat, doctors have wondered whether changes in fatty acids could be involved in multiple sclerosis (MS), a disease in which the myelin sheath is destroyed. The rate of MS seems to be increasing all over the world. This has coincided with decreased intake of essential fatty acids and increased intake of total fat.

Dr. Roy Swank was one of the first who pioneered the concept of an MS treatment based on dietary fat. He reported statistics showing that countries with the highest rates of MS also tended to have the highest rates of saturated fat consumption. High saturated fat intake commonly also means low intake of omega-3 fatty acids. Dr. Swank's pioneering work covered thirty-four years. Many thousands of patients have benefited from his dietary recommendations to modify fat intake.[3]

The Swank program involved:

- Saturated fat intake of no more than ten grams per day.
- Daily intake of forty to fifty grams of polyunsaturated oils.
- Avoidance of margarine, shortening, and hydrogenated oils.
- One teaspoon of cod liver oils daily (although other fish oils may be preferable)
- Consumption of fish three or more times a week.

The success of Dr. Swank's program coupled with knowledge that myelin is made of fat has encouraged many doctors to study the role of essential fatty acids in MS. When scientists studied the white matter of the brains of people with MS, they found a marked reduction in neural fatty acids such as arachidonic acid and DHA. They also found low levels of omega-3 fatty acids in blood and almost no omega-3 fatty acids stored in fat tissues.[4]

Does MS Susceptibility Begin in Childhood?

Doctors have wondered for many years whether events of early life played a role in susceptibility to MS. In 1994, physicians looking into the infant-feeding histories of people with MS met with some surprise. Those who developed MS were much more likely to have never been breast-fed or to have breast-fed for only a very short period compared with people who did not develop MS.[5] Remember that breast milk contains far more of the vital brain fats than cow's milk and formula, and that until 1997, formula has contained no DHA whatsoever. If MS is associated with early bottle-feeding it may be because the nervous system may not have received enough DHA at a critical period. This dietary influence may have influenced development of MS in someone with genetic susceptibility.

While at the Department of Neurology and Neurosurgery at Russian State Medical University in Moscow, I had numerous in-depth discussions with Dr. Yvgeny Gusev, President of the Russian Society of Neurology and Academician of the Russian Academy of Medical Sciences. His group had studied the risk factors to developing MS in Norway and Russia. They observed that consumption of meat in childhood and low fish consumption were key risk factors in the development of MS.[6] If this association proves to be true, it may be because the high DHA content of a fish-based diet protects the brain from autoimmune attack later in life. This idea is supported by experimental evidence that goes back many years with animals.[7]

Why Eskimos Don't Get MS

These findings are more plausible when you remember that Eskimo people seem to be protected against autoimmune attack and toxic injury to the nervous system by their high consumption of EPA/DHA-containing seafoods. They seem to be uniquely resistant to developing MS. At this time, the most logical explanation is that the high omega-3 fatty acid content of their diet protects them and argues further for a role of fatty acids in MS.[8,9,10]

MS Treatment with Fatty Acids

Several different treatment trials have been conducted using essential fatty acids in MS. Some have supplemented with omega-6 fatty acids while others with omega-3 fatty acids. The results of these treatments have been mixed.[11] This may be because of experimental design and failure to account for the full balance of fatty acids. Generally, people with MS who begin dietary changes early in the disease benefit most.

David Perlmutter, M.D., a neurologist from Naples, Florida, has used dietary management in multiple sclerosis for many years. He states that, "Balancing essential fatty acids is one of the most critical tools in my treatment of patients with MS. Using a low saturated fat diet that is enriched with gamma-linolenic acid from primrose oil and an omega-3 rich supplementation program has helped many of my patients. The key is to intervene early in the disease."[12]

PROTECTING AGAINST BRAIN ATTACK

Brain attack is a term doctors now use to describe stroke since the abrupt change in blood supply to the brain is much like that which occurs in a heart attack (when the heart's blood supply is abruptly interrupted). Brain attack includes a list of problems in which blood supply to the brain is altered for a brief or prolonged time.

While there are many dietary and lifestyle factors that put one at risk for having a brain attack/stroke, essential fatty acids have been found to play a role as well. In 1995, men who suffered strokes were compared with men who were stroke-free. Doctors found that for every .13 percent increase in blood ALA, there was a thirty-seven percent *decrease* in risk of stroke.[13] In other words, as the level of this omega-3 fatty acid improved in blood, the risk to stroke went down. In another study, doctors found that as vegetable consumption increased, the risk of having a stroke decreased.[14]

It is not entirely surprising that increasing the intake of fruits and vegetables lowered the incidence of stroke. Consuming some (green leafy) vegetables naturally increases the intake of omega-3 fatty acids, while eating fruits and vegetable increases antioxidants, trace elements, and other nutrients. Consuming more fruits and vegetables tends to reduce the intake of meat and other sources of saturated fat (as a percentage of their total calories).

In one study, people who ate at least two fish meals per month (high in EPA and DHA) had a sharply reduced risk to first-ever stroke and a reduced risk of brain bleeding. People who ate more than four meals of meat per week had an *increased* risk of all strokes combined.[15]

Anyone who has had a heart attack is subsequently at greater risk to having a stroke. In a group of people who had already suffered a heart attack, those who were told to eat fish two to three times weekly had a thirty percent reduction in death rate during the next two years, compared with those making no dietary fat changes.[16]

Fatty Acids and Risk Factors for Brain Attack

Doctors have identified a number of factors that place you at greater risk to having a stroke. These include:

- High blood pressure
- Atherosclerosis (narrowing of blood vessels by plaque)
- Diabetes
- Elevated cholesterol
- Alcohol consumption
- Smoking
- Heart rhythm problems (atrial fibrillation, etc.)

In all of these categories, essential fatty acids factor into the equation. For example, blood pressure is consistently lower in people who consume fish regularly.[17,18] In atherosclerosis, blood fats are often elevated while omega-3 fatty acids are low. In diabetes, omega-3 fatty acid levels are commonly abnormal along with an increase in lipid peroxides (rancid fats in the blood). Elevated cholesterol is often associated with low intake of omega-3 fatty acids.

Alcohol consumption is known to deplete important neural fatty acids as well as block the enzymes that form neural fatty acids from their precursors. Smoking may indirectly have an effect on fatty acids because cigarette smoke contains powerful oxidants and free-radicals that can deplete antioxidants and damage neural fatty acids. Vitamin C is especially affected, being much lower in smokers than nonsmokers.[19]

On the final point of arrhythmia, there may even be evidence that fatty acids have an impact. Atrial fibrillation, ventricular fibrillation, and other arrhythmias can cause inadequate amounts of blood to be delivered to the brain. They may also contribute to heart attack and stroke. It is well known that omega-3 fatty acids have a powerful impact on nerve conduction. In addition to being a pump, the heart is also an electrical organ. Nerve impulses are what precede contraction of heart muscle. There are now studies suggesting that essential fatty acids, in particular omega-3 fatty acids, can influence arrhythmias of the heart and visibly affect the electrocardiogram. Fish oil supplementation was even shown in one study to reduce arrhythmia in a group prone to this abnormality.[20,21]

As we age, the blood supply to the brain gradually declines. As shown in Chapter Three, this process often begins early in childhood and is tied closely to our intake of essential fatty acids. One means to preserve the brain's blood supply throughout life is to make sure fatty acid balance is adequate from beginning to end.

MIGRAINE HEADACHE

Migraine headache is also thought to be related to changes in the brain's blood vessels. Since essential fatty acids strongly affect messengers that influence the brain's vessels, some doctors believe that supplementation with fatty acids might be helpful in migraine. A group of fifteen people suffered from severe migraine headaches that did not respond to medication. Supplementation with EPA and DHA significantly reduced their headache severity and frequency.[22] Another group of people with severe migraine were given fish oil for a period of six weeks, after which they were given a placebo. While on the fish oil, migraine intensity and frequency was significantly reduced in five of the six people.[23] Fish oil may not be the ultimate solution to migraine headache, but these studies hint at a possible role for fatty acids. More likely, what's needed is a balance of fatty acids and their cofactors. Magnesium is among the critical minerals helpful in migraine.

DO FATTY ACIDS AFFECT BRAIN TUMORS?

In 1996, while speaking at a conference on brain injury, I had the privilege of spending several days with New York neurosurgeon Mehi Domacescu, M.D. When I asked him what has been his most striking observation of the past twenty years in his field, he quickly remarked, "the dramatic increase in brain tumors." Despite advances in detection, surgery, and radiation therapy, the survival rate for many brain tumors remains less than one year. Doctors aren't entirely sure what causes these tumors, which makes devising treatment strategies difficult.

Following my conversations with Dr. Domacescu I began wondering whether essential fatty acid imbalance might be associated with development of brain tumors. Then I reviewed the research of Dr. Douglas Martin and his colleagues, who studied the fatty acid content of the most prevalent of the brain tumors, malignant glioma. His group found that the DHA content of malignant glioma was only one-half the level found in normal brain tissue used for comparison.[24] Not only was DHA low, but linoleic acid (LA) was much higher in malignant tissue compared with non-malignant tissue. Other researchers have similarly found elevated LA and low DHA in various types of brain tumors.[25,26]

Martin's group has observed that fatty acid therapy may augment current therapies. They state that, "Dietary supplementation with PUFA [polyunsaturated fatty acids] has been demonstrated to alter the PUFA composition of not only normal brain tissue, but also that of intracerebrally implanted brain tissue. Indeed, intravenously administered fatty acids were more rapidly incorporated into the implanted tumor cells than the normal brain tissue. This ability to alter glioma cell PUFA composition might lead to an enhancement in the susceptibility of glioma cells to anticancer therapy."[27]

Could balancing fats and oils prevent or treat brain tumors? The answer will likely come as more doctors ask this very question.

LIFE IN THE STORM: FATTY ACIDS AND SEIZURE DISORDERS

Since seizures are associated with electrical problems in the brain, it is tempting to wonder how fatty acids might affect this disorder. Dr. Sidney Baker reported on one case of a child with seizures who also had patches of dry lusterless skin on his cheeks. Remember, such skin changes are common in fatty-acid imbalance. Dr. Baker began treatment with flax seed oil in an effort to correct the skin problem of the child's face. He had no particular aim to correct the seizure disorder with essential fatty acids. However, Dr. Baker observed that as the boy's skin problem improved his seizures also began to subside.[28]

Was this a case of brain-fats being too low? Could low brain-fats have affected the electrical activity of the boy's brain? It is hard to say for sure based on only one case. However, a recent article in *Medical Hypothesis* suggests that *febrile* seizures may be a result of certain messengers (IL-1) that are produced as a result of fatty-acid imbalance. The authors state that, "Diet supplementation of omega-3 fatty acids appears to offer an effective preventive therapy against febrile seizures that is less harmful than conventional prophylactic [preventive] methods."[29] There is also evidence that specific *saturated* fatty acids significantly improve some seizures.

Seizures may also be made worse by using certain fatty acids. This is why it is important to understand the individual's biochemistry before supplementing such a serious disorder. For example, it has been known for some years that evening primrose oil, a source of GLA, made seizures worse in some people. This likely occurred because the person's body was primed to convert GLA into arachidonic acid. In this state, the body would be making the wrong messengers. If a doctor were to use GLA in such a condition, he or she would need to pay attention to the factors that cause arachidonic acid formation.

Seizures involve a complex array of factors so I don't wish to offer fatty acids as a simple solution. Indeed, we don't really know much at all about fatty acids and seizures. Yet our growing knowledge of the importance of fatty acids in the brain may lead to some important breakthroughs in helping people with seizure disorders.

DISEASE OF THE EYES AND VISION PROBLEMS

In Chapter Two, I noted that the retina has the highest concentration of DHA of any tissue in the body. DHA balance in pregnancy, infancy, and adulthood may be crucial to developing and maintaining peak visual function. Beyond maintaining healthy vision, several specific disorders of the eyes may benefit from DHA supplementation. One in particular, retinitis pigmentosa, seems to have a close association with DHA.

Retinitis Pigmentosa

Retinitis pigmentosa (RP) is a group of hereditary disorders in which the retina progressively degenerates. The most common signs are increasing night blindness and loss of peripheral vision. Drs. Dennis Hoffman and David Birch measured the DHA levels of people with RP and found DHA levels to be forty percent lower than normal. None of the RP subjects had DHA levels comparable to people without visual problems. On further analysis, they also found that DHA levels correlated closely with retinal function as tested by the electroretinogram. The lower the DHA level, the poorer the retinal function.

It seems that people with RP have a block in the conversion of dietary alpha-linolenic acid to DHA. Therefore, LNA levels build up while DHA levels become too low. Because of this, it may be necessary to provide DHA directly in order to improve function to the retina or prevent further degeneration. Hoffman and Birch conclude, "Dietary supplementation with DHA would bypass several of the biosynthetic and transport steps and may restore blood levels of DHA to normal regardless of the specific mechanism impaired in the disease. It now becomes important to consider the potential for early nutritional intervention in patients with XLRP [X-linked retinitis pigmentosa]."[30]

Another condition characterized by degeneration of visual cells is Usher's syndrome, an inherited disease that leads to blindness. In this condition, DHA levels are found to be abnormally low as well.[31] We will see in Chapter Eleven that dyslexia, a visual disturbance associated with learning problems, may also respond to essential fatty acids.

Because vision problems become more common as we age, providing the retina's chief fatty acid DHA, may be valuable step in prevention and maintenance of healthy vision. For some specific vision problems, balancing fats and oils may be a necessary part of restoring peak function.

ON PINS AND NEEDLES: DIABETES AND NERVE DAMAGE

A sensation of pins and needles running down the limbs occurs in a condition called neuropathy. Neuropathy refers to damaging changes that occur to nerves, which can result in pain, loss of sensation, and death to the structures that the degenerating nerves supply. While neuropathy can occur in numerous circumstances, diabetes is perhaps the most common condition associated with neuropathy. New knowledge suggests that diabetics have abnormalities in fatty-acid status that affects their nerves.

According to Melvyn Werbach, M.D., former professor at UCLA School of Medicine, evening primrose oil is the "best proven nutritional intervention" for diabetic neuropathy.[32] In one double-blind study, 360 to 480 mg of GLA daily showed significantly improved nerve function after six months to one year.[33] Diabetics are also commonly deficient in omega-3 fatty acids such as ALA, EPA, and DHA. In fact, supplementation with these fatty acids has been shown to improve function of insulin receptors and improve the health of diabetics. In addition to fatty acids, nutrients that may be important include vitamins B12, B1, and B6.[34] Dr. David Horrobin, one of the pioneers in the field of fatty acids in medicine, recently found that a combination of GLA, EPA, and DHA worked best to correct symptoms of diabetic neuropathy.[35]

SCIATICA AND OTHER PAINFUL CONDITIONS OF THE LARGE NERVES

The sciatic nerve is called a peripheral nerve because it travels outside the spinal column. Since the nerve is one of the largest in the body and subject to its requirement for fatty acids, one wonders whether fatty acid consumption might cause the nerve to be especially sensitive or susceptible to interference. Neurologist Jean-Marie Bourre found that when you change the dietary balance of omega-6 and omega-3 fatty acids you can dramatically alter the fatty acid makeup of the sciatic nerve in animals.

He states, "Our preliminary results have shown that when rats are fed a diet deficient in omega-3 fatty acids (peanut or sunflower oil), both peripheral nerve and muscle contain reduced amounts of omega-3 fatty acids [specifically DHA]."[36] This makes one ponder what years of fatty imbalance might do to a person's large nerves if, as we've seen, it has so profound an effect on the nerves of the brain.

Recall also, the girl from Chapter One who was hospitalized following an abdominal wound. She was given an intravenous formula imbalanced in essential fatty acids—a formula not that different from the one given to Dr. Bourre's rats. While on the n-3-deficient diet she developed numbness, pain in her arms and legs, trembling in her left arm, blurred vision, and had difficulty walking. When the omega-3 fatty acid alpha-linolenic acid was increased in the feeding formula, her nerve symptoms cleared up.[37] Again, this suggests that fatty acid imbalance can also affect the large nerves that travel outside the brain and spinal cord.

CEREBRAL PALSY

Cerebral palsy is a broad term that describes a number of different disorders of the brain that happen before age five. It includes a wide range of symptoms. It often occurs from events at birth, but may be closely linked to what happens during pregnancy. The rate of cerebral palsy is highest in premature babies and has increased significantly among low-birth-weight babies.

Since premature or low-birth-weight babies do not have the benefit of a continued supply of brain fatty acids from the placenta, some doctors have begun to wonder whether CP is, in part, due to deprivation of key brain fats such as DHA. According to Dr. Michael Crawford, the DHA levels of a baby born prematurely fall quickly to only one-fifth of the level of the placenta. Unless the child immediately begins to receive DHA there may not be adequate brain-fats to properly form the developing nervous system.[38,39]

Looking carefully at the fatty-acid status of any child with cerebral palsy seems to be an important step in fostering recovery. Supplementation with fatty acids may allow slow restoration of some functions and may lead to an improved quality of life.

STAYING MENTALLY SHARP THROUGHOUT THE YEARS: FATTY ACIDS, DEMENTIA, AND ALZHEIMER'S

Staying mentally sharp throughout life is something most people find an important goal. In fact, when adults are asked what they fear most as they mature the most frequent response is loss of mental sharpness. Dementia is the term used to describe the loss of mental function. There is new evidence that certain fatty acids may protect against development of dementia and that fatty acids may be useful in some people once dementia has developed.

For example, people with decreased blood levels of DHA had almost twice the risk of developing dementia over the next nine years than with those whose blood levels of DHA was high.[40] A Japanese study of dementia found that sixty-nine percent of those whose dementia was due to blood vessel problems improved while on DHA supplements (700-1400 mg daily). Those with Alzheimer's disease experienced improvement in cooperation, speech, depression, and other psychological symptoms.[41] Dr. Horrobin and colleagues showed that patients with Alzheimer's disease had abnormal blood levels of fatty acids. Those who received essential fatty acids plus antioxidants showed improvement that was consistently better than those not receiving fatty acids.[42]

People with Alzheimer's disease also suffer from damage to fatty acids in various regions of the brain.[43] While we are nowhere near understanding this disease, recent studies suggest that essential fatty acids are destroyed in the brain, antioxidants are low, and lipid peroxides are high.[44]

Phospholipid treatment has also shown some benefit. In a study of fifty-one Alzheimer's patients, researchers gave 100 mg of PS three times daily for twelve weeks. Those treated with PS showed improvement on several measures of cognitive function.[45] In addition, nutrients such as acetyl carnitine, aimed at improving energy production in the nerve cell, have shown promise as well.[46]

All of this work suggests that atention to brain-fats throughout adulthood may be a powerful way to ensure peak mental function as we age.

OTHER NEUROLOGICAL DISORDERS

Many other neurological disorders exist that show some relationship to fatty acids or response to fatty acid supplementation. Dr. Margarita Woodbury of Harvard Medical School has treated over seventy children with neurological disorders using some combination of fats and oils.

One of her case reports was published in the *Journal of the American College of Nutrition*. A four-year-old boy was brought to her clinic with severe irritability, mood swings, inattention, feces smearing, and finger slapping. He was delayed in his speech and language, had movement problems and loss of sensation in portions of his body, and was behind in almost all developmental milestones.

During the course of treatment, Dr. Woodbury recommended lecithin, choline, and fish oil (EPA/DHA). The boy's neurological and behavior problems improved dramatically to the point that he was able to be mainstreamed in school. She reports that the boy has since successfully completed second grade and "continues to do very well."[47]

Down syndrome is another condition that reveals the brain-fatty acid link. Down syndrome is a genetic condition characterized by an extra copy of chromosome 21. People with Down syndrome often suffer from learning problems and commonly go on to develop a dementia that is similar to Alzheimer's disease.[48] The extra chromosome causes them to make more of a usually-helpful enzyme called SOD that contributes to a tremendous amount of free radical stress in the brain. This results in a high level of lipid peroxides, or rancid fatty acids, in the brain. Because of this, antioxidant nutrients are depleted and fatty acids are depleted.

Dr. Charles A. Thomas, Jr., director of Pantox Laboratories in San Diego, California has found that their blood is indeed commonly low in vitamins A, E, and beta-carotene.[49] Dr. J. Alexander Bralley, director of MetaMetrix Medical Laboratory in Norcross, Georgia, has also been evaluating nutrient abnormalities in Down syndrome. He has found an emerging and disturbing pattern of low levels of altered fatty acids and elevated lipid peroxides. Elevated lipid peroxides reflects the high degree of free-radical stress to which people with Down syndrome are exposed, and suggests that damage to brain tissue may occur. Moreover, lipid peroxides suggest that vital essential fatty acids are being degraded and destroyed.[50] This suggests that in Down syndrome, balancing essential fatty acids and antioxidants can be critical to preserving brain function.

Dr. Donald Rudin, one of the first to recognize the important link between fatty acids and the nervous system, reported back in the early 1980s on many cases of neurological conditions that responded to fatty acid therapy. He reviews a long list of cases of illness in which omega-3 fatty-acid insufficiency appears to be at the core.[51]

BEYOND THE EVIDENCE

We now have evidence that brain-fats may play a role in several different neurological diseases. One limitation of our knowledge is that we have not studied many other conditions of the brain and nervous system with regard to fatty acids. If the hypothesis is correct that proper amounts of neural fatty acids must be present throughout life, it may be that many other neurological disorders share this problem of inadequate fatty acids.

In the following chapter, we will weave together some of the evidence and see how fats and oils might possibly affect intelligence.

CHAPTER 11

ENHANCING MENTAL, PHYSICAL, AND EMOTIONAL INTELLIGENCE

Stephen Hawking is considered one of the most brilliant physicists of our time and holds the prestigious faculty position at the University of Cambridge once held by Isaac Newton. Highly regarded for his insightful and provocative book, *A Brief History of Time*, he has risen to almost mythic status among the public, having conducted his work while suffering from a severely crippling neurological disease.[1]

While his mental intelligence is especially astute, Hawking has been confined to a wheelchair for nearly twenty years because of Lou Gehrig's disease, a nervous system disease also known as amyotrophic lateral sclerosis (ALS). ALS has impaired Dr. Hawking's ability to move his body and has so impaired his speech that he now must communicate via a voice synthesizer.

Dr. Hawking's brilliance, courage, determination, and insight have been an inspiration to perhaps millions of people. Yet the juxtaposition of Dr. Hawking's physical disability and his superior intellectual power seem contradictory. We might say that while he remains superbly gifted in the area of mental intelligence, Lou Gehrig's disease has compromised Hawking's physical intelligence. His body no longer has the ability to properly determine its place within its surroundings and is unable to move in response to its surroundings.

In his landmark book, *Emotional Intelligence*, Daniel Goleman describes a young man named Jason who was a straight-A student at Coral Springs, Florida high school. He was fixated on getting into Harvard Medical School and felt a perfect grade point average was needed. However, his physics teacher one day gave him an 80 on a quiz. This must have threatened the young man's dreams because he took a butcher knife to school and, in an attempt to exact retribution on his teacher, stabbed his teacher in the collarbone. The courts found Jason temporarily insane during the incident. Jason subsequently transferred to another school, graduated at the top of his class with honors, and had a 4.614 grade-point average—well beyond A+. However, it appears that Jason never apologized to his old physics teacher who nearly lost his life because of the knife attack.[2,3]

How is it that someone with the mental brilliance to achieve straight-As can descend into such chaotic emotional depths that he would jeopardize everything by such an attack? Further, does the fact that Jason showed no remorse, never apologizing to his teacher for the attack, imply anything about his emotional intelligence? Goleman argues that emotional intelligence is a form of intelligence equal to or greater than mental intelligence, and that emotional intelligence is actually a better predictor of success in life. One might conclude from Jason's experience that he had superior mental intelligence, but poor emotional intelligence.

Then there is the case of Zane, a gifted young halfback and an intense competitor. After a brilliantly played game, I asked some of Zane's teammates if he intended to continue playing football in college. They looked at me dumbfounded. The star quarterback responded, "Were it not for the girls doing all of Zane's homework, we could have never kept him on the team. Zane will never make it through college. He is just not very bright."

Zane had superior physical intelligence. He was able to react with catlike quickness, deftly evade tacklers, and retain his balance in the face of jarring contact. Yet, his mental intelligence was not on par with his extremely high physical intelligence.

DESCRIBING INTELLIGENCE

We are accustomed to thinking of intelligence only in terms of IQ tests. But the work of many scholars has shown that the standard IQ test is a very shallow estimate of the complexity of human intelligence. Harvard Professor Howard Gardner has been one of the most ardent advocates of a more complex assessment of our intelligence. In his landmark book, *Frames of Mind*, he asserts that there are at least seven key forms of intelligence all of which interact to determine our success in life.[4] Author Tony Buzan proposes twenty different kinds of intelligence.[5]

Daniel Goleman, Ph.D. weaves a provocative story of how people who are successful in life are more likely to be emotionally intelligent than merely intelligent in the traditional sense.[6] In fact, many who are gifted in IQ often sabotage their lives by their low emotional intelligence. Philosopher and scientist Rudolph Steiner proposed early in this century that there were twelve attributes reflecting what we might today refer to as intelligence.[7] The work of these and other individuals illustrates that the debate surrounding intelligence has been waged for some time.

It is not my intent to redefine intelligence nor to challenge the existing opinions of what constitutes intelligence. However, for the purpose of simplifying our discussion, I suggest we describe intelligence within three domains: mental, physical, and emotional.* If we are willing to entertain this view of intelligence it may allow us to better understand a theme that runs throughout the study of fats and the nervous system.

Some individuals with fatty acid imbalance suffer problems that primarily affect what we might call mental intelligence. Others suffer changes that impair sensation, movement, and more physical attributes. Yet others with fatty acid imbalance experience difficulty in areas having to do with emotional intelligence. Not surprisingly, there are individuals in whom one or more of these attributes are simultaneously affected.

---

*Of course all attempts to reduce our attributes into neat boxes are fraught with potential for failure. But this breakdown may be useful to make a point.

We don't have enough knowledge to explain why fatty acid imbalance affects different individuals so uniquely. Given the fatty nature of the brain, however, it seems quite logical that intelligence might be affected at every level. As you'll note below, the story of how fatty acids may affect us across the spectrum of our intelligence opens up tremendous possibilities to transform the lives of individuals.

MENTAL INTELLIGENCE

Mental intelligence might include those things we typically associate with intelligence. This would include items measured in the classic IQ assessment, even though its value and sensitivity has been hotly debated. Also included under the rubric of mental intelligence are such things as memory, ability to learn new tasks, ability to understand complex information, and ability to generate new ideas from existing information. While many genetic, social, family, environmental, and other factors influence this form of intelligence, we are beginning to recognize that there are also many nutritional factors that affect mental intelligence.

The Case of Jenny

Perhaps nothing illustrates the power of fatty acids on mental intelligence so profoundly as the case of Jenny. She had struggled with learning problems all through childhood. By age twelve she was in the fiftieth percentile of her class. Life was a daily struggle to understand because her memory was so poor. A simple task or sequence of tasks was difficult for her to comprehend because she was unable to remember the sequence long enough to complete the task. She had particular problems with reading, spelling, and math. By grade three, she was being teased by classmates as being "dumb" and "stupid." Rarely would she study on her own initiative. Early in her schooling a teacher cruelly told Jenny's parents, "You had better get a calculator for this girl because she's going to need it for the rest of her life."

Not content to accept the dire projection of this and other teachers, Jenny's parents transferred her to a private school. Though Jenny enjoyed her new surroundings, her academic performance did not change appreciably. Then, in 1996, Jenny was started on supplemental fatty acids in an attempt to get more of the fatty acid DHA into her body. It was hoped that this might eventually improve brain function and academic performance.

After almost one year on DHA, she had risen from the fiftieth percentile all the way to the eighty-fifth percentile. She is now excited by school, interacts more fully with her peers, and is buoyed by high self esteem. She also studies independently with little help from others most of the time. To the astonishment and delight of her teacher, she recently scored a ninety-four on a spelling test. In short, the present has been transformed, while the future is filled with potential.

Jenny's moving story is a mere hint at the potential that exists to change people's lives through nutritional intervention. While her transformation is uplifting, the prospect that fats and oils might alter mental intelligence in not entirely new. This was illustrated dramatically in 1993 when animals consuming inadequate amounts of omega-3 fatty acids had difficulty learning to avoid a threatening situation. The high omega-3 fatty acid group was 100 percent successful after only three or four attempts. In the group fed a low omega-3 diet success was only thirty to forty percent even after the twentieth attempt. The authors concluded, "This indicated that a deficiency in the brain DHA level resulted in a reduction in learning ability."[8]

Carol E. Greenwood, Ph.D., wanted to see what affect fat had on memory and performance. Some animals were fed diets in which they received 10 percent of their calories from fat, while others received forty percent of their calories from fat. The remainder were fed between ten and forty percent fat diets. Forty percent is similar to the fat content of the standard American diet, so it is a realistic reflection of the amount of fat many people consume. The results were pretty clear. Animals who were fed the high-saturated-fat diets had the lowest performance on memory tests. Those fed the diets lowest in saturated fat did the best.[9]

In another study, researchers wanted to learn whether DHA supplementation improved memory. Using a passive avoidance test they learned that DHA has a beneficial effect on memory and that the effect is related to the amount of DHA given.[10]

Observing animals has led to some interesting insights on how fat might affect things like learning and memory, but what does it hold for humans? Like the story of Jenny above, it turns out that the mental faculties of humans may indeed be affected by fat. One intriguing discovery was made by British researchers who found that eight-year-old children who had been breast-fed as babies had higher IQs than those who had been formula-fed as babies. We know that breast milk is high in the brain-fat DHA, in addition to ALA and GLA, while formula has until recently had none of these. Researchers speculated that DHA could be the determining factor that gave the breast fed children the advantage. They also acknowledged other factors could be at work.[11]

In another study, boys with lower omega-3 fatty acids in their blood were found to have more learning problems than those whose levels were normal. When teachers were asked to evaluate academic skills, "math and overall academic ability was lower in the lower omega-3 fatty acid group."[12] We would expect children to be affected by fatty acid imbalance because their brains' are still forming. However, it appears that fatty acid imbalance may affect the cognitive function of adults as well.

Dr. Edward Siguel, of Boston University School of Medicine reported on several people who had laboratory evidence of fatty acid insufficiency. One had been suffering from long-term memory impairment and other vague mental impairments. Another had been suffering from psychiatric disease with mental impairment. What is interesting about both of these cases is that when alpha-linolenic acid was added to correct their fatty acid imbalance, their "memory and mental abilities improved."

Siguel contends that a large percentage of the population is deficient in fatty acids and derivatives critical to the nervous system. He remarks, "The chronic abnormal levels of DFA3s [derivatives of omega-3 fatty acids] could account for a significant proportion of mental impairments. While we spend billions to find a genetic cause or miracle drugs, we are overlooking the most common reason for mental impairments, a nutritional deficiency of the very long chain PUFAs [polyunsaturated fatty acids] that are the building blocks for brain function."[13]

Dyslexic individuals are well known to have defects in their retinas and in the brain processing of visual information and, as a result, experience unique challenges to learning. Dr. B. Jacqueline Stordy has studied adult dyslexics for the effect of DHA. She has found that, "DHA supplements given to dyslexics can also be associated with improvements in reading ability and behavior. These reports are anecdotal and subjective, but more formal studies are in preparation."[14] Additional fatty acids such as ALA and GLA may also be important in dyslexia.[15]

PS, PC, and Memory

Phosphatidylserine (PS) and phosphatidylcholine (PC) are phospholipids that contain essential fatty acids within their structure. Both have been used to enhance mental capacity. To date, there are over thirty-four human studies on PS, most of which have evaluated the role of PS in improving brain function. Some of the studies evaluated the effect of PS in people with impaired memory, behavior, personality, and concentration. Others studied the effect of PS in slowing mental decline in aging adults. In almost all cases, PS supplementation showed some benefit over placebo. In some trials, the results were highly significant.[16]

In one study of PS, a subgroup of people with memory impairment showed dramatic improvement following twelve weeks of PS supplementation. Using a parameter called Name-Face Recognition, researchers found that those taking PS improved an average of two points. On this scale, that is equivalent to "rolling back the clock" by nearly twelve years. A person of age sixty-eight might therefore experience an improvement of memory comparable to that of a fifty-six-year-old. This effect was not seen in all subjects, but was notable in those who were initially more memory impaired.[17]

In another study by the same group, subjects with mild memory impairment were studied for the effect of PS on ability to maintain concentration and overall improvement in cognitive status. A total of five functions were measured. PS supplementation was shown to provide benefit in four of the five functions tested. While the previous study showed PS benefit to those with more significant impairment of memory and cognition, this study showed benefit to those with mild impairment as well.[18]

The hippocampus is an area in the brain strongly related to the function of memory. With age, there is a gradual decline in receptors for a substance called nerve growth factor (NGF) and a decline in the number of dendrite connections within the hippocampus. This is one reason memory declines with age. It would be ideal if we could stimulate NGF and it appears that certain brain-fats may do just this.

When PS was given to laboratory animals there was an increase in NGF receptors and an apparent *increase* in production of NGF. In test tube experiments, PS directly stimulated NGF production.[19,20]

For many years, phosphatidylcholine (PC) has been used to enhance various aspects of mental intelligence. In disorders such as Alzheimer's disease or even the age-associated decline in mental function, decreased availability of choline is believed to play a role. M.I.T. researcher Dr. Richard Wurtman suggests that when inadequate choline is provided in the diet, the brain may actually cannibalize the phosphatidylcholine from its own neural membrane in order to obtain enough choline to make the neurotransmitter acetylcholine.[21,22]

This brief review of the evidence offers support for the idea that fatty acid balance is important in forging and maintaining what we might describe as mental intelligence. It goes a step further and suggests that specific phospholipids, which contain fatty acids, provide another element of support for mental intelligence under certain circumstances.

PHYSICAL INTELLIGENCE

Our bodies perform their complex physical tasks by integrating sensory and motor functions. Sensory functions involve the impulses that come into the brain that tell us about our surroundings. Pain, pressure, temperature, touch, vision, smell, and hearing are among the sensory functions. Sensory nerves relay back to our brains the position of our head, our arms, our legs, our fingers, and our toes. Our physical intelligence requires constant input about where our bodies are in space and how the movement of our millions of mucle fibers integrate. The motor cortex and the motor neurons generate the impulses that move our muscles in co-ordinated fashion so that we are able to interact with and manipulate our environment.

Because fats and oils so profoundly affect the structure of nerves and the brain as a whole, they have the potential to significantly affect the sensory and motor integration that allows our bodies to move intelligently in the world. In this regard, fatty acids may be said to affect our physical intelligence.

By our definition, we might say that multiple sclerosis involves a breakdown in physical intelligence. MS can affect many different regions of the brain, which dictates the nature of the symptoms an individual might suffer. We saw in Chapter Ten, that essential fatty acid imbalance may precede the development of multiple sclerosis and that fatty acid supplementation may improve the health of people with MS.[23]

We also saw how fatty-acid supplementation improved the paralysis and tremors of a forty-eight-year-old man. He was able to write, button his shirt, tie his shoes, and perform complex movements—things he was unable to do prior to supplementation with DHA. In addition, there was the case of the young boy who was unable to sit up under his own power and rarely walked on his own. He improved following DHA supplementation. One might argue that the physical intelligence was enhanced in each of these individuals. Their bodies became more capable of orienting themselves in space and moving within their surroundings.

The opening story of this book was noteworthy because, in addition to struggling with aggressive outbursts, Andrea suffered from problems with fine motor control. This makes delicate movements clumsy and difficult. We might say in her case as well that her physical intelligence was compromised. This was corrected by fatty acid supplementation.

The second story in Chapter One reviewed the case of a young girl who developed numbness of the hands and feet, loss of sensation, leg pain, blurred vision, tremors of the arm, and decreased vibration sense. Frequent episodes of weakness left her unable to walk for ten to fifteen minutes at a time. All of these may be thought to affect her physical intelligence, her ability to fully integrate her body within its surroundings. These changes were caused by fatty acid imbalance and were corrected by increasing the intake of alpha-linolenic acid, thus balancing the omega-6 to omega-3 ratio.

We have even seen in clinical practice individuals who suffered from neurological abnormalities characterized by something called hyperreflexia. Your tendons contain sensory cells that provide a constant stream of information to your brain about where your body is in space. In many ways, they are critical to our physical intelligence. When the doctor strikes just below the knee cap with a reflex hammer she is attempting to understand your deep tendon reflexes, or the status of the tendon sensors. This gives information about what is happening in your peripheral nerves or more deeply within your brain.

Excessive deep tendon reflexes (hyperreflexia) typically reflect one of many possible problems in the brain, usually a disease state. The term upper motor neuron lesion (UMN) is used to described one major category of brain disorders that might produce hyperreflexia. Doctors have now observed cases in which excessive deep tendon reflexes have been restored to normal following essential fatty acid supplementation.[24,25]

We are clearly only at the beginning of a new, exciting frontier. While far more work needs to be done, I believe we have enough evidence to suggest that, in certain individuals, fatty acid imbalance may compromise physical intelligence. As the story unfolds, it may become clear that fatty acid imbalance has the capacity to affect the physical intelligence of almost *any* individual. In most cases, fatty acids are likely not the sole nutritional factor nor the sole factor affecting brain function in general. Yet they are so fundamental to the brain's structure that they cannot be overlooked.

EMOTIONAL INTELLIGENCE

Psychologist Jack Block, at the University of California at Berkeley, has described a concept called "ego resilience," which shares many qualities with Goleman's picture of emotional intelligence. Extending from Block's definition, emotionally intelligent individuals would be socially poised, outgoing, cheerful, gregarious, not prone to fearfulness or worried rumination. They express their feelings appropriately (rather than, say, outbursts they later regret); they adapt well to stress. They have a notable capacity for commitment to people or causes, for taking responsibility, and for having an ethical outlook; they are sympathetic and caring in their relationships. Their social poise easily lets them reach out to new people: they are comfortable enough with themselves to be playful, spontaneous, and open to sensual experience. They rarely feel anxious or guilty.[26]

In essence, emotional intelligence is a complex mixture of qualities that allow us to function in healthy, creative ways in our relationships and within our surroundings. It allows us to cope with stressful circumstances and helps us find creative solutions to the myriad challenges that face us throughout life. As we reflect on the way in which fats and oils influences our behavior it seems reasonable to suggest that they affect our emotional intelligence as well.

Consider, for example, the numerous studies and case examples from Chapter Nine exploring the affect of fats and oils on development and treatment of depression and other affective disorders. Individuals who suffer from mood disorders, especially those that are chronic in nature may not have the emotional resources available to cope with their world in an optimum way.[27]

Consider also those with attention deficit hyperactivity disorder (ADHD). They are plagued with distractibility, impulsivity, and excess nervous energy. They are commonly hypersensitive to their surroundings and often have difficulty controlling their impulses. People who suffer from this disorder may act inappropriately on impulses, in a repetitive pattern that leads to harsh discipline, which only heightens the tension in their already tense lives. Quite often their condition is not due to their fundamental family dynamics, but to a basic biochemical imbalance.

When we revisit the work presented in Chapter Nine we see that ADHD may have associations with fatty acid imbalance.[28,29] Drs. Sidney Baker and Leo Galland were both once with the Gesell Institute of Human Development and work extensively with ADHD. They have observed that ADHD can often be successfully managed by supplementation with primrose oil, flax oil, or fish oil—sources of GLA, ALA, and EPA/DHA respectively.[30,31] Balancing fats and oils in some of these individuals may have a profound effect on emotional intelligence for years to come.

The importance of fatty acids in emotional intelligence was further reflected in a study of college students who were followed from the end of summer through final exams. Final exam period is an extremely stressful time for students and stretches their coping skills to the brink. Many suicides and violent and hostile acts have been committed by distraught students during finals. I recall a college classmate who jumped off the Washington Avenue bridge at the University of Minnesota during finals. Another attacked a pizza delivery man with a knife. Though finals are stressful for everyone, some students fare worse than others.

There are certainly many psychological and social variables that come to bear on how students cope with such challenging times. Yet, there may be nutritional factors that are important. A group of college students was given a daily supplement of the fatty acid DHA beginning in August and continuing through final exam periods. Doctors wanted to study a measure of behavior called external aggression—aggression toward another person. It is often accentuated when a person is under stress. Students who received DHA supplements for the entire fall period through finals displayed far less external aggression than those not taking supplements of this fundamental brain fatty acid.[32]

I believe this study, if corroborated by further research, holds an important message. Someone who is perpetually aggressive or circumstantially aggressive would not be viewed as emotionally intelligent. However, the low emotional intelligence may not be based solely on the grounds of their habitual patterns. It may boil down to fundamental biochemical pathways that are influenced by nutrition, in this case, fatty acids. We see, time and time again in clinical practice, the adult or child whose aggression, malaise, or inability to cope are changed once brain metabolic pathways are modified with nutrition.

Consider the pregnant mother, for example. She may go through life emotionally stable and healthy. Within days or weeks of delivery of her child, however, a deep dark melancholy descends upon her life. Feelings of unworthiness, thoughts of suicide, worries that she may injure her baby, an entire range of feelings complicate this period of postpartum depression. It is as though the emotionally intelligent woman is adrift in an irrational sea of fear, uncertainty, and melancholy. While the cause of postpartum depression has not yet been discovered and is undoubtedly complex, we saw in previous chapters that the blood levels of long-chain fatty acids fall precipitously during pregnancy and lactation.

Recall the words of Drs. Joseph Hibbeln and Norman Salem who comment on the subject of declining fatty acids in pregnancy: "This relative maternal depletion of DHA may be one of the complex factors leading to increased risk of depression in women of childbearing age and in postpartum periods."[33]

A final example of the possible effect of fats and oils on emotional intelligence regards women with premenstrual syndrome (PMS). It is well known that some women who suffer from PMS have tremendous mood swings and find coping with life very difficult. Women who are emotionally healthy, stable, creative, and insightful may experience such dramatic changes in mood during the premenstrual period that their judgment, perception, and response to the world around them becomes altered. Courtrooms have even ruled in favor of women who use PMS as a defense in cases of assault or automobile accidents.

British studies have shown that GLA (from evening primrose oil) can relieve about ninety to ninety-five percent of women's premenstrual tension. Doctors have found that evening primrose oil alleviates symptoms of about two-thirds of women not helped by anything else. GLA probably works to alleviate the mood swings and other symptoms of PMS by modifying the messengers called prostaglandins. These prostaglandins have direct effects on mood and may also affect fluid accumulation within the brain, which affects function.[34]

In his book, *Emotional Intelligence,* Goleman has a chapter titled "Temperament is Not Destiny," in which he shows how many patterns of our emotional matrix that we associate with temperament are more malleable than we might believe. As we grow and develop, our specific temperamental qualities are met in various ways by our parents, teachers, and others in our lives. This strongly shapes the way in which our temperaments manifest and express. Goleman suggests that careful nurturing throughout childhood and attention to needs at critical windows of development may allow children the best chance for developing emotional intelligence that will carry them into adulthood.

From what we have seen so far of the ability of fats and oils to transform the lives of individuals, I think it can be said that these nutrients also have the ability to shape temperament and aid in building a brain that supports the development of emotional intelligence. Like Goleman, I believe there are crucial developmental windows and that the right balance of fats and oils must be present in order to make the most of the neural potential with which a child is endowed at birth. Failure to adequately meet these windows may disadvantage a child and influence her life into adulthood. Properly meeting these periods may give every opportunity for optimal emotional intelligence that lasts a lifetime.

THE SEAT OF INTELLIGENCE: WHERE IS IT?

The preceding discussion, that fatty acids affect the brain and thus affect intelligence, is founded on one very bold assumption: that the brain is the seat of intelligence. The view of the brain as the seat of intelligence is not, however, shared by all cultures nor by all scientists. Some cultures are known to confer the sense of "I" to various body parts, for example, the heart or the abdomen. When noted anthropologist Margaret Mead was asked where in her body her consciousness resided, she replied, "Why, all over!" So much of our daily bodily activity goes on without any conscious awareness that one wonders whether there is an intelligence at work that orchestrates the trillions of "decisions" that happen each moment of our lives. Do the cells that secrete our hormones have intelligence? Do the white blood cells that travel to the site of infection have intelligence? If all of this activity goes on without our conscious awareness, does intelligence then reside within every cell within our body?

Larry Dossey, M.D., has addressed this question in some depth and remarks, "Our concept of our brain as the center of thought may be utterly spurious, a kind of chauvinistic cerebralism which will not bear the scrutiny of our new knowledge. Far better, perhaps, to regard the entire body as a brain—if by brain we mean the site of human thought."[35]

If the entire body and its host of cells is regarded as intelligent, does this not cast doubt on the idea that fatty acids affect intelligence by affecting the brain? Perhaps, but consider that every tissue and organ in your body is made up of cells. Within each cell, the complex web of interdependent systems operate to make our hormones, create energy, communicate with one another, reproduce, repair, and sustain life.

Recall from Chapter Two, that most cells within the body (except, for example, bone cells) are surrounded by a flexible membrane that is composed primarily of fat. Essential fatty acids are critical structural and functional components of these membranes. Recall also the work of Sidney Baker, M.D., and his colleagues at Yale. They calculated the total surface area of our lipid membranes to be roughly equivalent in size to ten football fields. This translates into a vast sea of essential fatty acids.

If we summarize how fatty acids affect the "intelligent" operations of cells, we see that they affect:

- Energy production
- Gene expression
- Control of inflammation
- Control of immune function
- Cell membrane fluidity and ability to change shape and migrate through tissues
- Cell membrane permeability—what gets in and out of the cell

- Cell communication
- Detoxification of harmful substances and waste

Consider also that instructions are sent from the brain that govern the trillions of cellular activities that occur beneath our conscious awareness. In turn, the cells relay signals to the brain that inform the brain of what is happening in the complex symphony of bodily activity. This aspect of cell "intelligence" is dependent upon nerve-cell integrity which, as we've seen, is highly dependent upon fatty acid balance.

Taken together, it seems clear that fatty acids are central to the *structure* of every cell and central to the *function* of every cell. If we assume that intelligence resides not only within the brain, but within every cell of the body, we must conclude that cell intelligence and therefore body intelligence is powerfully affected by essential fatty acids.

BUILDING INTELLIGENCE

As we contemplate the role of fats and oils in intelligence we must realize that intelligence is a complex set of phenomena. It requires fundamental attributes provided by our genetics and then careful nurturing provided by hours and hours of repetition, use, and integration. It is further influenced by our social environment, our relationships, and such things as chemicals, foods, nutrients, toxic metals, physical activity, and the entire web of our existence. In building intelligence we must take all of these things into consideration.

Presently, we have more questions than answers regarding how and to what extent fatty acids affect intelligence. But the evidence we have tells us that fat forms the architecture upon which our brains are built and the architecture upon which our cells our built. More than perhaps any other nutrient, fatty acids have the capacity to affect the very essence of who we are.

PART IV

GETTING THE BRAIN-FATS YOU NEED: FOOD AND SUPPLEMENT GUIDE

CHAPTER 12

FEEDING THE BRAIN, MIND, AND BODY: THE BEST FATS AND OILS

As we better understand the brain's critical dependence on specific fats and oils, we move beyond the commonly-held view of fats/oils as mere sources of flavor or calories. Fats and oils now rise to a level in our consciousness that place them at the very top of our dietary and health considerations. Selection of the appropriate fats, oils, and supplements, therefore, becomes one of the most important tasks we undertake in pursuit of optimal wellness.

THE *SMART-FAT DIET*

In the following two chapters, I will describe the basic principles of what I call the *Smart-Fat Diet*. Recall that *Smart-fat* refers to two basic concepts:

The intelligent (*smart*) use of fat. Don't under consume or over consume fat, while balancing total fat with adequate essential fatty acids. Don't become fat-phobic, become *fat-smart.*

The use of fats that foster intelligence (fats that make us *smart*). Consume fatty acids needed in brain function that may build mental, physical, and emotional intelligence. These are fats that influence the intelligent operations of the brain and body.

The *Smart-Fat Diet* is not list of recipes, but is a set of principles and concepts that guide us in our use of fats and oils.

EATING WITH INTENT AND PURPOSE

While I have provided a model of how fat affects the brain based on biochemistry and neuroscience, I would never propose that our eating habits be centered on so mundane a concept. The value of food to our bodies goes well beyond simple nourishment and bio-chemistry. In many cultures, eating is seen as a meditative experience in which our full intent is focused on eating. As some of the wisdom keepers have said, "When you eat, eat. When you sleep, sleep. When you walk, walk." If we do things with focus and in-tent, the richness of the experience is more likely to come through. When we eat with the television on, while reading the paper, or when driving to our next appointment, we lose the full value of what the eating experience might bring to our lives.

The ultimate goal in creating a diet that best serves your needs is to have foods that are visually appealing and flavorful, while pro-viding the optimum balance of nutrients. In my view, food gather-ing, preparation, and eating should all be undertaken with great consideration. It should be gathered with foresight and insight, with consideration of its origins, balance, and harmony. It should be prepared with loving intent, using methods that best preserve the balance of elements. It should be eaten with gratitude, slowly, with full consideration given to its presentation and surroundings.

Without these things, the process of providing nourishment becomes mechanical. It may provide basic nutrition, but it lacks some of the more ephemeral qualities that have been so cherished through the ages.

FOOD VS. SUPPLEMENTS

In this chapter, I will focus on the food sources of the brain-fats and give you some ideas about their preparation. I always believe that food is where healing begins. Supplements can be extremely helpful and often necessary, but I believe they are never a substi-tute for creating a vibrant, balanced diet. On the other hand, ours is a fast-paced world filled with meals cooked or consumed "on the run." For practical reasons, daily supplementation of specific fats and oils is probably a necessity for many people. They may find it difficult to obtain the proper balance of oils through food. For people suffering from illness, supplements may be the only way to obtain the quantity of specific fatty acids needed to bring about healing.

BALANCE OF TYPES IS CRITICAL

As you've read this book, you may have gathered the impression that omega-3 fatty acids are more important than omega-6 fatty acids. The story I have woven may give this impression because most modern diets contain far too much omega-6 and far too little omega-3. Because of this, my thesis has focused on the need for omega-3 and the need to reduce omega-6.

In reality, we need a balance of omega-6 and omega-3 fatty acids. Excessive omega-6 intake can lead to trouble, while excessive omega-3 intake can present its own set of problems. There are even cases in which excessive omega-3 consumption has led to symptoms such as ringing in the ears, or tinnitus. In practice, most people will end up increasing their omega-3 intake, while decreasing their omega-6 intake. Others may need to increase specific forms of both omega-6 and omega-3 oils. You must come away from this book with this very important point. Balance of essential fatty acids is critical. We don't want to go overboard on any particular fatty acid.

PROTECTIVE NUTRIENTS

Whenever you increase your intake of unsaturated fatty acids, be aware of the fact that they are extremely sensitive to oxidation or damage. This is also true when the fatty acids exist in your body. Increasing antioxidant food and nutrient consumption is a *must* when fatty acid intake is increased. Vitamin E in the form of a mixed tocopherol is central among these. Additional antioxidants such as those described in Chapter Six are also important. Always consume antioxidants nutrients in a balance.

FINDING THE FUN IN A SMART-FAT DIET

As you contemplate changing to a diet more rich in brain-fats, realize that a diet should not be bland, dull, boring, nor an exercise in deprivation. Food is one of greatest gifts on earth that goes well beyond its mere ability to nourish and sustain. Food should stimulate the senses and be a source of blissful experience and splendor. I believe that we can have both if we are creative. I also believe that if we eat well, there is a little room for some decadent fun. The key is to know what you are dealing with and what you are up against.

VEGETARIANS

Recall from previous chapters that vegetarians are commonly low in DHA. This is thought to be because vegetable-based diets provide no preformed DHA. Vegetarians thus must rely on their conversion of ALA to DHA—a process that may be quite inefficient in some people. This makes use of dietary supplements containing DHA very important in vegetarians. Because supplements are now available that are not derived from fish, but from algae, vegetarians should have no philosophical objection to supplementation.

Vegetarians also commonly choose margarine over butter to avoid use of an animal product. I believe the use of margarine for this philosophical reason is a biochemical mistake because of the trans fatty acids present in margarine.

OBTAINING QUALITY OILS

Many techniques used in modern processing and preparation of oils for sale to the public result in damage to essential fatty acids, the presence of trans fatty acids, and residue of solvent extraction. The food oil industry has a history of providing products to the marketplace based on ease of shipping and storage. Health considerations have often been secondary to shelf-life concerns. In order to derive the most benefit from consuming oils (and avoid making things worse) attention to quality is very important.

Below is a list of suggestions that will allow for selection of oil products of the highest quality and purity. Also included is a list of suggestions for storage that will maintain that quality once it's in your kitchen.

1. Attempt to get your oils from whole foods where possible. This means consuming fish, walnuts, flax seed meal, sesame seeds, or other products rather than just consuming the oil. Recall that foods such as flax seed contain, in addition to fatty acids, compounds such as lignans with many significant health benefits.

2. Use oils that are certified organic. Many industrial and agricultural chemicals are fat-soluble and tend to concentrate in the oil portion of plants and animals. Organic products do not contain chemicals applied in the growing process and commonly have a nutrient density greater than non-organically grown products.

3. Use oils that are stored in dark bottles. Essential fatty acids are subject to rancidity when exposed to light. Dark bottles prevent this from occurring. Grocery store shelves are filled with oils in clear glass or plastic bottles, which only invites light to further oxidize the fatty acids.

4. Oils with a high content of unsaturated fatty acids spoil more easily with increasing air exposure. Oils should be kept covered.

5. Oils with high unsaturated fatty acids spoil more easily when exposed to warm temperatures. Keep them refrigerated at all times. Those high in monounsaturates like olive oil, need not be refrigerated. Oils rich in saturated fat, such as coconut oil or ghee, also need not be refrigerated.

6. Use oils that are *unrefined*. Oils processed in this way are most closely related to the original product and are least likely to contain damaged fatty acids. Refined oils are commonly extracted with toxic solvents and processed at temperature above 400 degrees F.

7. Oils should be cold-processed, expeller pressed. Look for a statement on the label regarding the temperature at which the oil was processed. It should ideally be between 86 and 110 degrees F.

The Omegaflo process used by some companies protects the oils during processing and results in a high quality oil product.

8. If you taste an oil that seems bitter, it has probably become rancid. Consuming these oils should be avoided.

COOKING WITH OILS: THE WET SAUTE METHOD

Cooking with high temperatures is how many oils are damaged. One way to avoid this is to primarily cook with oils that contain mostly saturated fat such as coconut oil, ghee, or butter. Oils containing mostly monounsaturates such as olive oil are also fine for cooking. However, the taste of many other oils such as sesame are delightful. One way to preserve their integrity while still enjoying their taste is to "wet sauté." In this method, place a small amount of water in the pan or skillet and heat until just below boiling. Add the food you desire and sauté. As the food becomes cooked, add a small amount of oil. This shortens the time the oil is in contact with the heat, yet preserves the flavor in the food. Oils should not be heated to the point of smoking.

IN SEARCH OF OMEGA-3

Since omega-3 containing foods are less common in our diets and more difficult to find, I've provided a brief guide to these foods separately. Following this discussion is an overview of the various oils used for consumption and their fatty-acid content.

Foods Containing Omega-3 Alpha-Linolenic Acid

Oil	Approximate Percentage ALA
Flax	58
Hemp seed	25
Pumpkin seed	1-15
Canola	10
Soybean	7
Walnut	5
Wheat germ	5
Chia	30
Kukui (candlenut)	29
Green Leafy Vegetables	variable

The following oils are good oils, but they contain little or no omega-3 fatty acids. Therefore, they should always be balanced with an omega-3 containing oil.

Unrefined safflower   Unrefined sunflower
Sesame   Rice bran
Evening primrose   Black currant seed
Borage

Foods Containing DHA

Cold water fish are the richest sources of DHA (and EPA). Some species contain more than others and the content of an individual species varies somewhat from fish to fish. The DHA content of farmed vs. wild fish can be considerably different depending upon the feed given to commercially raised fish. Consuming fish two to three times per week is an excellent way to increase omega-3 fatty acid content. In general, the fish containing the highest amounts of DHA include:

Salmon   Mackerel
Herring   Sardines
Trout   Eel
Plankton, algae   Anchovies
Bluefin   Albacore tuna
Caviar

Warm water fish like orange roughy, red snapper, and swordfish do not contain much DHA. EPA/DHA is also found (though in much smaller quantities) in fresh water fish such as:

Lake trout   Haddock
Walleye   Northern Pike
Carp

Chicken and Eggs as a Source of DHA

Chicken meat may contain DHA if the bird has been raised on a high omega-3 fatty acid feed. Chicken eggs also naturally contain

DHA. However, the amount is highly dependent upon what the chicken is fed. Dr. Artemis Simopoulos showed, for example, that Greek eggs (grown by feeding fish meal to laying hens) contained 6.6 mg of DHA for every gram of yolk, while regular supermarket eggs contained only 1.09 mg of DHA.[1] Since DHA is very susceptible to oxidation, cooking or overcooking chicken eggs may destroy some of this delicate fatty acid.

CHOOSING THE BEST OILS

In choosing oils for internal use always remember to use organic oils or seeds. Seeds tend to concentrate pesticides and other undesirable substances. Moreover, many steps in the commercial processing of oils can add toxic residue and remove healthful component such as lignans. Below is a discussion of the fats and oils commonly used in food preparation, in health promotion, and in treating illness. They have been subdivided into those that contain omega-3 fatty acids, those predominant in omega-6 fatty acid and omega-9 fatty acids, and those predominant in saturated fat. To maintain adequate levels of brain-fats, I believe it is important to balance the intake of omega-6 and omega-3 fatty acids in an approximate one to one ratio (1:1). For most people living on modern diets, initially consuming more omega-3 oils may be necessary.

OILS CONTAINING OMEGA-3 FATTY ACIDS

Below is a discussion of oils containing omega-3 fatty acids. These oils also contain omega-6 and omega-9 fatty acids in variable amounts.

Canola Oil

Canola is a coined term that refers to the oil derived from a hybrid of the rapeseed plant. This plant belongs to the *brassica* family, which includes cauliflower and mustard. It is sometimes referred to as rapeseed oil, however, canola and rapeseed oils are fundamentally different. Rapeseed is high in a fatty acid called erucic acid, once believed to be associated with toxicity to heart cells. Modern canola oil contains less than two percent erucic acid, a level not associated with clinical problems.

Canola oil is the most widely used oil in Canada and its use in the United States is growing rapidly. Common commercial forms may be overly processed. Some canola is organically produced and some companies who use canola oil in their products routinely test to ensure that oil with chemical residue is not used. Canola oil is used in salad dressing, mayonnaise, and vegetable oil spreads. It is not recommended for high-temperature cooking because of its omega-3 fatty acid content. Do not heat above 120 degrees F. The omega-6 to omega-3 ratio of canola oil is a very desirable 2:1.

Fatty acid content: n-3 = 10%; n-6 = 24%; n-9 = 60%.*

Chia Seed

Chia seeds are second only to flax seed in their content of omega-3 ALA. They are commonly used in baking and used in various dishes. A common food used in Mexico to promote endurance and improved energy.

DHA-Containing Oil

Commercial supplements are now available that contain DHA as the primary fatty acid. Currently available forms are derived from algae grown to specifically concentrate DHA with no EPA. If one wishes to specifically increase DHA levels (without increasing EPA levels), a DHA supplement is the most desirable route. It is also preferable for people who have concerns about possible toxic residue in fish oil. Dosages typically range from 100 to 200 mg per day. When used in the treatment of specific disorders, higher levels may be recommended. Since DHA is the most highly unsaturated of the fatty acids commonly used, it is also the most subject to ran-

---

* Note: Published values of fatty acid content of oils may vary based on the plant species, growing region, and other variables.

cidity. Always store it in the refrigerator or freezer. Take additional vitamin E and a mixed antioxidant formula when consuming added DHA. DHA is never used in cooking or in food preparation.

There is currently only one over-the-counter product that contains straight DHA from a plant source (Neuromins, 100 mg DHA).

Flax Seed Oil and Flax Seed Meal

Flax seed oil is the richest source of the omega-3 fatty acid alpha-linolenic acid at roughly fifty-seven percent. Its omega-6:omega-3 ratio is a very desirable 0.3:1. Flax seed oil can be used daily as a reliable source of omega-3 fatty acids. One should never use flax oil for cooking or baking. Flax oil *must* be refrigerated and will only last for two or three months once opened. However, it can be stored in the freezer to increase its shelf life.

Ground flax seed or flax seed meal is another way to increase omega-3 intake. This not only provides fatty acids, but lignans as well. Some clinicians shy away from using flax meal with pregnant women because it can have a laxative effect in high doses. If this is of concern, using flax oil during this time is desirable.

Flax seeds can be used in baking. Some bakeries now add flax seed or flax seed meal/flour to their bread and muffins to increase the omega-3 content. There has been some concern that adding flax seeds to baked good might increase the formation of rancid fats. However, recent studies suggest that the level of rancid fats is not increased by baking with flax seeds.[2] Baking with flax *oil* is an entirely different matter and, as noted above, should be avoided. Flax seeds are very hard and chewing them does not easily liberate the oil. Grinding flax seed fresh with a coffee grinder each morning is another way to obtain the benefits of the flax fatty acids. Be sure to grind only for the minimum period of time needed to break up the seeds.

Fatty acid content: n-3 = 57%; n-6 = 16%; n-9 = 18%.

Fish Oil

Cold water fish such as salmon, mackerel, herring, and sardines are rich sources of EPA and DHA. At least two servings of cold water fish per week should be considered. Even at this level, however, getting the ideal amount of EPA and DHA may be difficult. Dietary supplements may be needed to reach desired levels of DHA. For vegetarians, DHA supplements derived from algae are available.

Fish oil supplements may not be suitable for infants and small children for at least two reasons. First, the brain has no apparent requirement for EPA. In attempting to get DHA from fish oil, too much EPA ends up being consumed. Second, EPA is known to displace arachidonic acid from cell membranes. While this may be desirable in an adult who has accumulated too much arachidonic acid over his lifetime, it is not desirable for many children. In fact, fish oil ingestion in infants has produced modest decreases in growth.[3]

Premature infants are especially at risk to brain hemorrhage. They should not consume an EPA-containing oil because EPA can increase bleeding times. A solution to providing adequate DHA in infants is to use a supplement containing only DHA.[4]

Fish or algae-derived oils are never used for cooking because of their high unsaturate content. They should be stored in the refrigerator or freezer. Fish oil intake has been shown to increase the level of lipid peroxides in the body, which seems to be related to increased need for vitamin E. Thus, vitamin E levels should be increased whenever taking fish oils.

Fatty acid content: Varies between species.

Hemp Seed Oil

Hemp seed oil is not widely used, but is among the richest sources of alpha-linolenic acid (25%). Hemp seed oil has been added to various natural foods to increase their omega-3 content.

Walnut Oil

Certain varieties of walnuts provide modest amounts of omega-3 fatty acids. However, commercial walnut oils are often overly processed and undesirable. Organic walnut oil can be obtained by special order if desired. Walnut oil should not be used for cooking. Consuming whole walnuts is another means to increase the omega-3 content of the diet.

Fatty acid content: n-3 = 5%; n-6 = 51%; n-9 = 28%.

Wheat Germ Oil

Wheat germ oil contains modest amounts of omega-3 alpha-linolenic acid (up to 5%). In addition, it contains a fatty alcohol octacosanol. Octacosanol has reportedly been shown to increase stamina and endurance by increasing oxygen utilization. More recently, octacosanol and other fatty alcohols have been shown to help restore neural function in various brain disorders such as stroke, brain injury, and coma.[5] Octacosanol derived synthetically from non-wheat germ sources is not the same as that used in the clinical studies of Dr. Thomas Cureton. These studies were carried out using a concentrated wheat germ source produced by the Viobin Corporation.

OILS CONTAINING OMEGA-6 AND OMEGA-9 FATTY ACIDS

Almond Oil

Organic almond oil has a sweet, desirable taste. It can be used to lightly saute in food preparation. However, most commercial almond oils in the United States are overly processed. Thus, almond oil is primarily used as a topical oil in massage.

Fatty acid content: n-6 = 26%; n-9 = 65%.

Borage Oil

Borage seed oil is a rich source of the omega-6 fatty acid GLA. GLA is often used to increase the body's production of the messenger family PGE1. It is very helpful in conditions where the enzyme that converts the body's fatty acids is not working adequately. Borage oil contains approximately twice the level of GLA as oil of evening primrose. This oil is not used for cooking. It is usually sold in soft-gel capsules. Typical doses range from one to six perles daily depending upon age. Higher doses are often used under guidance of a health professional. GLA should be used with caution in people with tumors.

Cottonseed Oil

The principal fatty acids are linoleic, oleic, and palmitic acids. Cotton is heavily treated with pesticides making cottonseed oil a poor choice for internal use. Nevertheless, cottonseed oil is widely used in processed foods such as chips.

Fatty acid content: n-6 = 48%; n-9 = 23%.

Evening Primrose Oil

Evening primrose oil is a rich source of the omega-6 fatty acid GLA. GLA is used to encourage formation of the messenger family of PGE1. Primrose oil is available as a supplement and is not generally used in cooking. It is usually sold in soft-gel capsules. Typical doses range from one to six perles daily depending upon age. Higher doses are often used under guidance of a health professional. In one study of diabetic neuropathy, up to twelve perles per day of evening primrose oil were consumed daily with beneficial results. Use with caution if tumors present.

Fatty acid content: n-6 GLA = 9%.

Hazelnut Oil

Hazelnut oil is preferred as one of the finest gourmet oils by some of the world's top chefs. Jeff Woodward, a Minneapolis nutritionist, chef, and macrobiotic cooking educator, feels that hazelnut oil is one of the finest cooking oils available. It is similar to olive oil in that it contains a high proportion of monounsaturates (omega-9 fatty acids). While it contains no omega-3 fatty acids, the low proportion of omega-6 unsaturated fatty acid yields a low likelihood of rancidity when used in cooking.

Fatty acid content: n-6 = 15%; n-9 = 76%.

Olive Oil

Olive oil is one of the most reliable cooking oils and is one of the most healthful oils for general use. Its high oleic acid content makes it very stable for cooking. It is rich in antioxidants and phytonutrients. Extra virgin organic olive oil should be sought since many commercial brands are solvent extracted.

Olive oil contains only marginal amounts of omega-3 fatty acids, but the high oleic acid content may aid in incorporating omega-3 fatty acid into membranes. However, its many general health benefits make it perfectly suited to any dietary style that includes omega-3 fatty acids from other sources.

Fatty acid content: n-6 = 8%; n-9 = 82%.

Peanut Oil

Peanut oil is very high in monounsaturates making it stable for cooking and frying. Commercial peanuts are grown on soil in which herbicides and pesticides are often used, making most peanut oil undesirable for consumption. *Organic* peanut oil should always be sought. The high levels of lignoceric and behenic acids also make peanut oil an undesirable oil for widesread, regular use.

Fatty acid content: n-6 = 22%; n-9 = 60%

Pistachio Oil

Pistachio oil is considered among the best "gourmet" oils and is highly valued among some of the top chefs. Its high oleic acid content makes it quite stable for cooking at medium temperatures. Pistachio seeds are valued as a tonic in traditional Ayurvedic medicine. It contains no omega-3 fatty acids and does not contribute to the brain-fat pool.

Fatty acid content: n-6 = 31%; n-9 = 54%.

Pumpkin Seed Oil

Pumpkin seed and some squash seeds contain omega-3 alpha-linolenic acid in addition to their omega-6 and omega-9 fatty acids. This benefit is offset by the fact that obtaining organic pumpkin seed for commercial use is difficult. Growing your own pumpkins and consuming the seeds is one way to take advantage of this delicious and nutritious food, with its nice balance of fatty acids. Pumpkin seeds and pumpkin seed butter make wonderful snacks if you are able to find an organic source.

Fatty acid content: n-3 = 1-15 %; n-6 = 60%; n-9 = 20%.

Safflower Oil

Safflower oil is high in omega-6 fatty acids. A "high oleic" safflower oil is currently available, which may be a better choice. There are various opinions regarding the value of safflower oil for use in foods. In general, its high omega-6 content places it low on the list of oils desirable on a Smart-fat diet.

Fatty acid content: n-6 = 79%; n-9 = 13%.

Sesame Oil

Sesame oil is used extensively in Asian and Middle Eastern cuisine. It has a long history of safe use and can be processed at low temperatures, which is desirable to prevent rancidity. Sesame oil is also high in lignans, one of which is called sesamin. These lignans appear to block the enzyme that makes excess arachidonic acid. Thus, sesame oil may be helpful in cases where this enzyme is too active. Sesame can be used for low-temperature frying. It also contains a naturally-occurring compound called sesamol that imparts antioxidant protection. Since sesame oil is fairly high in linoleic acid, its intake should always be balanced with omega-3 oils.

Fatty acid content: n-6 = 41%; n-9 = 49%. Also contains phosphatidylcholine.

Sunflower Oil

Sunflower oil was once highly valued by the ancient Incas. Because of its high linoleic acid content, sunflower oil contributes to an already high linoleic intake in modern societies. A "high oleic" sunflower oil is now available, which has a reduced linoleic content. This should be the only form used when the taste of sunflower oil is desired. In general, because of the fatty acid profile, sunflower oil is low on the list of oils considered beneficial on a Smart-fat diet.

Fatty acid content: n-6 = 69%; n-9 = 19%

FOODS PREDOMINANT IN SATURATED FAT

Butter

Butter is rich in saturated fat and contains no omega-3 fatty acids needed for the brain. The debate over whether butter is better than margarine has heated up recently because of growing concern about trans fatty acids in margarine. Almost without exception, the colleagues with whom I associate professionally agree that butter is a better choice than margarine. We also agree that butter intake should be kept to a minimum because of its high saturated fat content. It should be organic whenever possible to avoid the antibiotics and growth hormones used in commercial animal husbandry. If butter is used, a daily dose of essential fatty acids rich in omega-3 must also be used. Another alternative is to use ghee (See below).

Some people enjoy a spread made by mixing equal parts of softened butter with olive oil. Since it is a monounsaturated oil, olive oil is an excellent substitute. Flax oil can be used instead of olive oil in this mixture. Once mixed, however, the spread *must be refrigerated* or the flax oil will become rancid. Better yet is a mix containing two parts non-hydrogenated, unrefined coconut butter and one part flax oil (for omega 3).

Coconut Oil

Coconut oil is rich in saturated fat and contains no appreciable unsaturated fatty acids. Though it is a saturated fat, unlike butter which contains long-chain saturated fats, coconut oil is rich in medium chain triglycerides, which contain fatty acids of eight to fourteen carbons in length. *Non-hydrogenated* coconut oil has many health benefits and should contain no trans fatty acids. Coconut oil provides no omega-3 fatty acids. However, the lauric acid in coconut is helpful in some brain conditions and also possesses significant anti-viral activity.

Coconut oil is perhaps the best "high temperature" cooking oil for those who do not want to cook with animal products such as butter. It is very stable at high temperatures because it contains negligible amounts of unsaturated fatty acids.

Fatty acid content: n-6 = 1%; n-9 = 9%; saturated fat = 89%.

Ghee

When butter has had the milk solids removed it is referred to as ghee. Ghee is widely used in India and is valued in Ayurvedic medicine for its ability to enhance the *ojas*. By balancing the *ojas*, ghee has been observed to support physical and mental renewal. Ghee is an excellent cooking oil because it is high in saturated fat, fats that do not oxidize when heated to normal cooking temperatures. Ghee is one of the most highly regarded cooking oils in the world for the unique flavor it adds to almost any dish. It should be organic whenever possible to avoid the antibiotics and growth hormones used in commercial animal husbandry.

While ghee is an excellent cooking oil and possesses some healing properties, it remains a source of saturated fat that is devoid of EFAs needed by the brain. Therefore, when using ghee, remember that you must supply additional EFAs from another source.

Fatty acid content: n-6 = 30%; n-9 = 5%; saturated fat = 65%.

Margarine

I place margarine in the saturated fat category because many margarines are high in trans fatty acids, which behave much like saturated fat. Some companies have come out with margarines made from non-hyrogenated canola oil with other added elements. They may have lower levels of trans fatty acids, around fifteen percent. Since there are so many sources of wonderful oils that nourish the body, there seems to be no particular reason why anyone would choose margarine.

Fatty acid content: variable depending upon form.

AVOIDING FOODS HIGH IN TRANS FATTY ACIDS

In Chapter Seven, we reviewed the potential problems with consuming trans fatty acids. These altered fats are best left out of the diet. Common sources include:

French fries	Deep fried fish burgers
Cookies	Deep fried chicken nuggets
Candy	Deep fried mushrooms, cheese curds, etc.
Potato chips	Puffed cheese snacks
Tortilla chips	Corn chips
Cake	Doughnuts
Mayonnaise	Margarine
Shortening	Salad dressing (other than olive oil-based)

Oils for Use in the Smart-Fat Diet

Oil	Baking	Light Saute*	Applied Cold**	Contains Omega-3	Helps PGE1
Almond Oil	•	•	•		
Borage Oil			•		•
Canola Oil			•	•	
Chia seed	•		•	•	
Coconut oil	•	•			
DHA (from algae)				•	
Primrose Oil			•		•
Flax seed Oil			•	•	
Flax seed or meal	•		•	•	
Fish Oil			•	•	•
Ghee	•	•	•		
Hazelnut Oil	•	•	•		
Olive Oil	•	•	•		
Pistachio Oil		•	•		
Pumpkin Seed Oil			•	•	
Safflower Oil	•		•		
Sesame Oil	•	•	•		•
Sunflower Oil	•		•		
Walnut Oil			•	•	

* Use of low temperatures is generally desirable for all oils.
** Applied cold means that the oil can be applied after the food has been cooked or prepared.

PHOSPHOLIPID SUPPLEMENTS

Additional supplemental nutrients called phosphatidylserine (PS) and phosphatidylcholine (PC, a.k.a. lecithin) have been discussed at times in this book. These are fatty substances that contain fatty acids within their structures. Both have been found helpful in a variety of brain disorders and have been helpful in improving depression, memory, and cognitive function. A brief discussion of each is listed below.

Phosphatidylserine

Recall from Chapter Four, that phosphatidylserine (PS) is one of the structural molecules of nerve cell membranes. It is the major *acidic* phospholipid in the brain. PS is formed when the phospholipid complex combines with the amino acid serine. PS has several important related functions. It strongly influences the fluidity of nerve-cell membranes and is necessary for electrical activity in the brain. PS is vitally important (along with PE [phosphatidylethanolamine]) for the incorporation of membrane proteins, or receptors. Recall that membrane proteins are like the antennae bound to cell membranes. They are critical for the binding of neurotransmitters and, thus, nerve transmission. The fatty acids found in PS are critical to this function.

PS is generally found in one of two sources—soy and bovine. Most clinical studies with PS have been done using the bovine source. Bovine PS is essentially derived from purified cow cerebral cortex or spinal cord. This source of phospholipid is most likely to have more highly unsaturated fatty acids like DHA as part of its structure. The soy-based PS does not appear to have the same amount of highly unsaturated neural fatty acids as part of its structure. In addition, there are fewer studies using the plant source. However, one study using the plant source showed significant benefit in improving depressive symptoms.[6] Some reports from clinicians with whom I've talked suggest that the soy-based PS does result in clinical improvement.

Philosophically, I am more comfortable with the plant source of PS because of concerns over slow virus contamination of bovine PS. Virus contamination has not been shown to be a problem, but it remains a concern. Studies with PS have generally used doses in the range of 100 to 300 mg per day.

Phosphatidylcholine

Phosphatidylcholine (PC) has at least two important functions in the brain. First, it is a vital component of nerve cell membranes. Like PS, it is necessary for electrical activity in the brain as well as being needed to hold membrane proteins in place. Second, the choline portion of PC is used by neurons to manufacture the neurotransmitter acetylcholine. Neurons in the brain do not make their own choline, but receive it from the blood. Once they receive choline they manufacture acetylcholine. If the diet does not contain enough choline, this neurotransmitter is not produced adequately.

In disorders such as Alzheimer's disease or even the age-associated decline in mental function, decreased availability of choline is believed to play a role. Recall also the work of Dr. Richard Wurtman suggesting that when inadequate choline is provided in the diet, the brain may actually cannibalize the phosphatidylcholine from its own neural membrane in order to obtain enough choline to make the neurotransmitter acetylcholine.[7]

Phosphatidylcholine is usually derived from soy or egg. Its common name is lecithin and is available in supplemental form. Many commercial forms of lecithin have less than thirty percent PC. One should get a lecithin that contains over over thirty percent PC. Combination supplements containing PC and PS are also available.

FAT AND OIL SUPPLEMENTS TO KEEP YOUR BRAIN IN SHAPE

A basic supplementation strategy for improving intake of fatty acids in *healthy* people might include those listed below. Individuals with medical problems may consider a basic strategy to balance fats and oils. However, high-dose supplementation with any particular fatty acid should be undertaken with caution. Consultation with a health professional knowledgeable in fatty acid nutrition is advisable.

- ALA from flax oil: 1 to 3 teaspoons daily depending upon age.*
- ALA from flax seed meal: 2 to 4 teaspoons daily depending upon age.
- DHA from algae oil: providing 25 to 100 mg DHA daily.*
- Alternate source of DHA: Fish Oil—providing up to 200 mg EPA and DHA daily.* (Don't use with infants.)
- GLA from borage or primrose Oil.
- Vitamin E: 50 to 400 IU daily.

---

*The optimal intake of alpha-linolenic acid for healthy adults is estimated to be 800 to 1,100 mg per day. EPA/DHA intake is suggested to be about 400 mg daily.

- Mixed antioxidants
- Nutrients to boost mitochondrial energy. (See Chapter Six.)
- PC: 50 to 100 mg daily.
- PS: 50 mg daily
- Botanicals such as *Ginkgo biloba*.

Fatty acid supplements are now available that contain GLA, ALA, and other fatty acids in an approximate omega-6 to omega-3 ratio of 1:1. These would seem to be very good for general use, especially if they also contain DHA.

WE ARE ALL UNIQUE

While we all share vast similarities, each of us is unique in our history, genetics, lifestyle, dietary preferences, and life experience. As such, recommendations that attempt to fit us all into the same box may need to be fine-tuned for optimum benefit. The general description of fats and oils contained in this chapter allows for a general approach to *balancing* fats and oils. However, each individual's needs will be specific to his or her own set of circumstances. This requires that you proceed from a base of knowledge and then experiment with that which feels most comfortable. By listening to your body's needs you can gradually find a state of balance that nurtures you to optimum health. Some people may require the help of a trained professional or additional resources when beginning this journey. *Healing with Whole Foods* by Paul Pitchford (North Atlantic Books, Berkeley, California) is a valuable resource in this regard.

CHAPTER 13

BEWARE THE LOW FAT DIET: IN PURSUIT OF BALANCE

Because the average adult in affluent countries gets about forty percent of his or her calories from fat, we've been told to "cut out the fat" at almost every turn. Stroll through any grocery store aisle and the words "fat free" and "low fat" leap off the packages. Amble through the book store and you'll be confronted with volume after volume on low-fat, low-cholesterol diets.

Weight-loss programs of every form advocate losing weight by cutting fat, often down to ten percent or less of total calories. Many programs aimed at reversing heart disease advocate cutting fat to ten percent of calories. Fitness programs chide us to trim down by exercising and cutting out fat. In short, we've become a nation of fat-phobics. At the same time, the rate of obese and overweight Americans is growing.

While logical and well-intentioned, these low-fat/no-fat recommendations often fail to recognize the absolute requirement of the brain for essential fatty acids. Some people indeed must reduce their intake of total fat, but in doing so, must maintain appropriate amounts of unsaturated fatty acids to sustain peak brain performance. Failure to adjust our fat intake to achieve balance may lead to problems in the brain.

According to Charles Glueck, M.D., "the same low fat diet that ensures cardiovascular health will ensure brain health." He suggests that the diet needed to boost mental performance contain a mere ten to fifteen percent of calories from fat.[1] When Glueck makes these recommendations, I believe he is primarily focused on improving brain performance by keeping blood fats low, fats such as triglycerides and cholesterol. This approach to maintaining brain function is based on blood flow to the brain.

He may not be focused on the need for DHA in the brain, the need to balance messengers like prostaglandins, the need for essential fatty acid balance, or the specific need of individuals. He may be incorrect in stating that ten percent fat is good for the brain because this low level may not provide enough essential fatty acids for peak brain performance. In reality, we don't know.

Dr. Dean Ornish has shown that heart disease can be reversed, in part, by using a diet composed of ten percent fat. His dietary strategies are highly restrictive of fat. Mary Enig, Ph.D. suggests that our ancestors consumed diets very low in unsaturated fatty acids and recommends a thirty to forty percent fat diet with less than five percent as polyunsaturates.

William Connor, M.D., of Oregon Health Sciences University, suggests that a diet containing twenty percent of calories from fat is ideal for optimum benefit. He goes further, however, and states that forty percent of the *fat* should be in the form of essential fatty acids. Saturated fat should only compose about four to six percent of your total calories.[2] While we cannot be sure if Dr. Connor's recommendation is accurate, his recommendation may be more realistic because it emphasizes both the need for modest fat intake and essential fatty acid adequacy.

If one looks at the historical record, it is clear that fat intake varied widely around the world. Some groups consumed as little as ten percent of their calories from fat, while others like the Inuit people consumed as much as sixty percent of their calories from fat.

General recommendations may be helpful, but they often do not address the needs in special circumstances. For example, for an athlete in training, ten percent fat may not be enough to sustain energy needs. During pregnancy, fifteen percent fat may be far too low to sustain existing levels of fatty acids, not to mention providing adequate EFA for the developing fetal brain. An infant must get fifty percent of her calories from fat. A nursing mother must still maintain her high fat intake during the nursing period. Moreover, since the mother's DHA stores fall so far during pregnancy and lactation, it is probably wise for a woman to maintain a higher fat intake for some time after delivery.

An individual who regularly consumes alcohol may need specific fats such as GLA and DHA to compensate for the effects of alcohol on the brain. Someone with digestion or absorption problems may already be absorbing inadequate amounts of fat. Reducing fat intake to ten or twenty percent of calories without addressing their specific fat needs may not only reduce availability of brain-fats, but may restrict fatty acids needed to repair the digestive membranes themselves. Women attempting to bear a child may not be able to conceive or carry a child to term if they are fatty-acid deficient.

Additionally, low-fat diet recommendations do not take into consideration that we may already be the third or fourth generation that has gotten inadequate omega-3 fatty acids. We will see in the final chapter that fatty acid imbalance appears to be cumulative, meaning the dietary habits of our parents and grandparents influence our own nutritional status.

It may seem confusing, but I believe that doctors who make blanket statements about cutting fat intake do some people a disservice. Low fat diets across the board can benefit many people, but they have inherent risks for others. This is especially true if they tend to also reduce essential fatty acid intake. You don't want a diet that aggravates a nutritional deficiency.

In my opinion, the low-fat diet is a slippery slope unless it contains these elements:

- Tailored to your individual needs.
- Ensures that you get enough unsaturated fatty acids.
- Ensures balance of omega-6 and omega-3 fatty acids.

These are conditions with which most of the low-fat diet advocates would probably agree, especially if given the opportunity to review the evidence on fatty acids and the brain. There is no question that many people get too much fat in their diets. But we must be sensible in the way that we approach fat intake.

Another point also deserves consideration. When people reduce their fat intakes, they must naturally fulfill their caloric needs with something else. This generally ends up being either carbohydrate or protein. When carbohydrate is increased too high it may favor the formation of arachidonic acid and potentiate the inflammatory process. If one increases protein intake from animal products such as beef or pork, arachidonic acid intake is increased. This seemingly confusing, and somewhat oversimplified view merely urges that we be sensible about our balance of nutrients.

Below is a discussion of circumstances in which one should be cautious about a low-fat diet. Caution does not necessarily mean that a low-fat diet should be avoided. It merely means that the decision should be individualized and that the diet should maintain fatty acid balance.

Dangers for Children

Infants must get about fifty percent of their calories from fat. Within this there must be a substantial amount of unsaturated fatty acids. If you restrict fat intake in this critical age you may negatively affect development of the brain. Many infants consume large amounts of cow's milk, which is high in saturated fat and devoid of brain-fats. Some parents have attempted to provide a low-fat diet to their infants by feeding skim milk. This practice can also cause difficulty because if causes the protein to fat ratio to be too high for a child in this age range.

From age one to age two, the fat requirement of a child is still higher than that of an adult, so cutting out total fat is dangerous. Cutting out unsaturated fatty acids can be disastrous.

Dangers for Pregnant Moms

Low-fat diets should never be used by pregnant mothers unless specifically recommended by a doctor to achieve a specific goal. Even then, adequate fatty acids must be supplied to support brain development. Most American women already get too little of the unsaturated fatty acids needed for brain development. Further lowering fatty acids during pregnancy might lead to toxemia, premature delivery, growth problems, and risk to neurological or behavioral diseases in the child.

Dangerous Weight-Loss Diets

Many weight-loss diets significantly restrict calories including essential fatty acids. Remarkably, many overweight people find that as they increase their intake of essential fatty acids it is easier to lose weight. Any weight-loss program that restricts fat intake *must ensure that essential fatty acid intake is adequate.*

Vegetarians

Vegetarian diets can be of great benefit for many people. However, as we saw in Chapter Four, vegetarians tend to be low in DHA. This may be, in part, because of high consumption of omega-6 oils. A more likely explanation regards the fact that vegetarian diets contain no preformed DHA. They must rely on conversion of alpha-linolenic acid to DHA, which is an inefficient process. Vegetarians thus would not benefit from further fat reduction. They may, in fact, need to increase intake of certain fats.

Meat and Potatoes

The person who has been on a traditional American diet of meat and potatoes can certainly benefit from cutting down on total fat intake. However, these same individuals commonly consume very little of the omega-3-rich foods needed for peak brain performance. Cutting out the fat without increasing the intake of omega-3 fatty acids may further compromise health.

Dangers for People with Behavior and Mood Problems

While low-fat diets can help some people with mood and behavior problems, especially those whose triglycerides are elevated, it can aggravate the problem in other people. Recall that depression, aggression, violence, attention deficit, hyperactivity, and other behavior difficulties have been associated with altered fatty acid balance. Reducing total fat without attention to the specific fatty acid needs of each individual could further complicate such conditions.

Dangers for People with Neurological Disease

Some neurological disorders such as MS may improve when a low-fat diet is introduced. This has certainly been shown in the thousands of people who have benefited from the diet of Dr. Roy Swank. However, when specific essential fatty acids are added to the low-fat program, results are often enhanced. It is important to realize that in neurological disease nerve-cell membranes are being destroyed. In order for the body to repair these membranes it must have raw materials in the form of fatty acids. Once again, simply cutting out the fat in the diet is a short-sighted approach. Specific attention to the individual's needs is the only way to proceed, in my opinion.

I have visited hospitals and clinics in different parts of the world wherein certain fatty acids, fatty alcohols, and gangliosides are given in the treatment of stroke, brain injury, and other disorders of the brain. This is in keeping with the brain's need for fat to regenerate its neurons. Tailoring fat intake to the individual seems inherently more wise than merely restricting fat in such cases.

Difficult Kids in the School Setting

There is a general trend among childhood medical and nutrition advocates to reduce the fat content of children's meals. This is a worthy and desirable goal if undertaken with essential fatty acid balance in mind. However, if we look at the behavior and discipline challenges in schools and couple that with our new knowledge of how fats affect behavior, we cannot be simplistic about cutting the fat from childrens' diets. If we reduce total fat we must also ensure adequate amounts of omega-3 fatty acids and an adequate balance between omega-6 and omega-3 fatty acids.

VIOLENCE AND AGGRESSION

While high-fat diets certainly contribute to behavioral problems, it is important to recall the studies in which low-fat diets led to increased violent, aggressive behavior and social isolation. Additionally, some members of one study engaged in self-mutilation. A society with problems of aggression and violence, such as our own, can ill-afford to make dietary recommendations that might possibly aggravate the problem. In this regard, I believe we must temper our "no-fat, low-fat" recommendations and recognize the crucial role of fat in individuals and in culture. Those who engage in violent aggressive behavior commonly suffer from fatty-acid imbalance. Further restricting their fatty-acid intake may not lead them down a path of recovery.

GUIDES TO A LOW-FAT INTAKE: THE *SMART-FAT* DIET

Recall from the previous chapter that I introduced the term the *Smart-Fat Diet*. I believe we should do away with the term low-fat diet because it gives us the mistaken impression that all fat is bad—that we should keep fat intake "low." Low means different things to different people, even in the medical community. More-over, as we've just seen, low-fat diets are not suitable for everyone. However, a Smart-Fat Diet is suitable for everyone because it:

• Balances total fat with adequate essential fatty acids according to the needs of the individual.
• Uses fatty acids needed in brain function that may foster intelligent operation of the body's systems.

In general, the *Smart-Fat Diet* should contain the following considerations:

• Keep total fat intake around twenty to thirty percent. Higher or lower in certain circumstances.
• Reduce saturated fat intake when appropriate.
• Make sure your unsaturated fat intake is adequate, perhaps forty percent of total fat.
• Keep the omega-6 to omega-3 ratio between 1:1 and 3:1 if possible.
• Make sure it is rich in nutrients that help in the use of fatty acids: Mg, Zn, B6, B3, vitamin C.
• Never use unsaturated omega-3 fatty acids for cooking.

- Avoid trans fatty acids.
- Ensure that the diet contains antioxidant-rich foods that may help protect brain membranes.
- Use blood tests, where necessary, to fine-tune your specific fatty acid needs.

These changes will help us enormously in our evolution toward a more sensible relationship with fat. It will allow us to avoid the pitfall of the high-fat diets so common today and ensure that we don't further deplete our brain fatty acids in the process.

THE POWER AND THE POTENTIAL

The story of fatty acids and the brain confers great hope that we may be able to change the course of our individual lives and perhaps even society by making wise dietary changes. Attention to the brain's fatty acids may also allow us to raise our level of function to new heights as we combine good nutrition with the vast knowledge about human potential we've amassed.

Awareness, however, always leaves us with a choice. Should we choose the path of inattention and show little regard for these influences, the outcome may be of evolutionary proportions. In the final chapter, we will learn what evolutionary biology has revealed about the brain's nutrient needs and what other species may be teaching us about our future.

CHAPTER 14

SHAPING OUR FUTURE, LEARNING FROM OUR PAST

As we further unlock the mystery of how fatty acids affect the brain, we are faced with evidence that compels us to wonder where the dietary habits of our culture are leading us as a species. Many lessons about our potential future lie woven into the fabric of history and the evolution of other species. When added to the current picture described in this book, it leads to some very provocative conclusions.

Our first glimpse into this world comes from knowledge of how fat affects brain size. Evolutionary biologists have for years studied the brain-to-body size of mammals. Though there are notable exceptions, it seems that as the body size of animals increases, brain size decreases. Scientists have further discovered that the fats needed to make a large brain are different from those required to make a large body. For example, saturated fat is good for rapid body growth, but poor for rapid brain growth. Unsaturated fatty acids have a less dramatic effect on body growth, but are critical for brain growth.

Cows, for example, provide milk to their calves that is very high in saturated fat and almost entirely devoid of brain fats such as DHA. Accordingly, a calf grows dramatically in its first months of life, but its brain grows very slowly. In the adult cow, the brain is pitifully small compared with its body. Human milk, on the other hand, is rich with highly unsaturated fatty acids, but low in saturated fat. Human babies grow very slowly, but their brains nearly triple in size during the first year of life.

Dr. Michael Crawford, of the Institute of Brain Biochemistry and Human Nutrition, has reviewed the influence of fat on brain size in his book, *Nutrition and Evolution*. Referring to the rapid growth of large animals and their fat use he states, "the capacity to produce long-chain neural lipids does not keep pace and their concentrations [of DHA] in tissues falls away as animals get bigger: consequently the brain loses out. Hence there is a universal contraction of the size of the brain relative to the body it serves, as well as a loss of large functional zones [of brain]."[1]

This may have relevance to our own situation since, in many cultures, there is solid evidence that body size has increased significantly.[2] This trend coincides with increasing consumption of beef, dairy products, and total calories. These foods are high in saturated fat and generally devoid of certain neural fats.

If we follow Dr. Crawford's logic to its conclusion we must wonder: Is it possible that the increased body size of people consuming high-fat diets has occurred with a price? Is it possible that the price has been paid by the brain itself? To date, there is no specific evidence showing that human brain size has decreased. However, we may be paying the price in the form of functional changes of the brain described elsewhere in this book.

This argument grows more interesting when we look at what happens to animals deprived of critical brain fats over generations. At the National Institutes of Health (NIH), doctors fed animals diets deficient in omega-3 fatty acids from infancy, throughout development, and through adulthood. This practice is fairly common in people consuming a standard modern diet. As a result of this diet, there was a fifty percent drop in the brains of one of the most crucial brain fats (DHA) by adulthood. The next generation of animals fared even worse. Their brain DHA levels had fallen by ninety percent in both infancy and adulthood.[3]

Similar results have been obtained by other researchers.[4] If the same holds true for humans, it suggests that the consequences of consuming inadequate brain-fats does not end with ourselves, but is passed to our children and our grandchildren. Moreover, it appears that the effects may be magnified in each subsequent generation. As noted previously, those of us alive today may already be part of the second, third, or fourth generation raised on diets low in essential brain-fats.

Returning to the dietary trends of humans we'll recall that ancient diets contained a ratio of omega-6 to omega-3 fatty acids estimated to be roughly 1:1. Today, that ratio is more on the order of 30:1.[5] Dr. Rudin's suggestion that our omega-3 fatty acid intake has fallen by over eighty percent over several generations leads one to conclude that we may be experimenting with the human brain in much the same way the NIH scientists modified the animal brains over successive generations.[6]

Dr. Crawford has made another curious observation about the evolution of animals. He suggests that animals such as apes lost brain capacity as they ran out of foods rich in omega-3 fatty acids, especially DHA. They, in effect, devolved.

He writes, "Biochemical analysis of the tissue arachidonic [AA] and docosahexaenoic acid [DHA] content of savannah species shows clearly that all large species have more or less run out of [DHA]. They are effectively essential fatty acid-deficient, and particularly so of [DHA], which provides a tested mechanism for determining the loss of brain capacity and function." He goes on to add this very important conclusion: "Nutrient limitation induced the loss of relative brain capacity as the animals evolved with faster growth rates and larger bodies. They outstripped the ability to produce the neural nutrients."[7]

Dr. Crawford, and his colleague from the University of Toronto, Dr. Steven Cunnane, challenge existing theories of how the human brain rose to a level of complexity beyond other species when they state, "man did not necessarily develop a larger brain, rather other species may have, in relative terms, lost brain size. The loss was also associated with a low availability of [long-chain polyunsaturated fatty acids], and particularly DHA."[8]

Their observations are remarkable, for if they are right, evolution of a complex brain is not driven so much by random selection as by nutrient availability. In other words, the raw materials available to the brain via the diet may be one of the key factors that determines the size and complexity of the human brain.

If other species lost brain capacity because they ran out of DHA and other omega-3 fatty acids, with what did they build their brains? It appears that a replacement fatty acid from the omega-6 family became one of the key building blocks for the brains of these species.

This draws us to a pattern that repeats itself with humans as well. It appears that when brain fats such as DHA are not present in adequate amounts, the brain must create a substitute to form its structure. According to Dr. C. D. Stubbs, "when cells are deprived of sources [of DHA] in the diet the cell will tend to produce the nearest fatty acid (in terms of unsaturation and chain length) that is possible, even if the fatty acid is from the omega-6 series."[9] The replacement fatty acid from the omega-6 family is often DPA, the same fatty acid found in greater amounts in mammals with smaller brain sizes. DPA has been found to increase with:

- Alcohol consumption.
- Essential-fatty-acid insufficiency (especially DHA and ALA).
- Trans fatty acid intake.
- Excessive omega-6 intake.

DPA has also been found to be elevated in conditions such as depression and attention deficit hyperactivity disorders.

Crawford and Cunnane make a very important point when they ask, "As all land-based species lost relative brain capacity as they evolved larger bodies, how is it that *Homo sapiens* broke that rule and did the opposite by evolving a larger and larger brain?"[10] In their writing, they conclude that ancient humans did not break the rule, but retained their access to the sea where they were able to gather omega-3-rich foods needed by the brain.

Hidden within his question seems to be a challenge, however, that we cannot break the rule. It is true that as we fill up on fats that promote large body growth that we may deprive ourselves of fats that promote brain growth. If the brains of animals such as apes declined as they ran out of omega-3 fatty acids, we may likewise be unable to escape the fate of our current decreasing intake of neural fatty acids. If the observation of Crawford and Cunnane is indeed a rule, our future may be tied to our intake of essential fatty acids.

If their assessment is correct, our culture has undertaken a bold and dangerous dietary experiment with consequences that might affect all of society. When we reflect on the evidence presented in this book and combine it with this view of the evolution of the brain, there is a sense of urgency. How do we avoid the fate of the animals who may have traveled this path over the centuries?

While evidence from the past and findings of the present give some cause for alarm, they also provide incentive to bring about change. The somber warnings of the decline of other creatures may spur us to recognize the powerful force of nutrition, not only on health, but on the evolution of our species.

Society currently grapples with medical and social problems that defy easy explanation. These new insights surrounding fatty acids and the brain suddenly give us a largely unexplored tool to improve the lives of individuals and, perhaps, even society. Dietary fat now emerges as a nutrient, not to be spurned or avoided, but to be revered and respected for its remarkable potential to transform our lives.

POLYUNSATURATED, MONOUNSATURATED, AND SATURATED FAT IN SOME COMMON FOODS*

Fatty Acid Content in Selected Fats and Foods

	g/100 g			
	Polyunsaturated	Monounsaturated	Saturated	Total fat
Fats and Oils				
Almond	27	66	7	100
Apricot kernel	33	62	5	100
Avocado	15	69	16	100
Babasso	2	15	83	100
Butterfat	3	31	66	100
Castor	3	96	1	100
Chinese tallow	0	27	73	100
Chicken fat	20	49	31	100
Cod liver	35	50	15	100
Cocoa butter	2	36	62	100
Coconut	1	7	92	100
Cohune	1	10	89	100
Corn	59	35	16	100
Cottonseed	83	9	8	100
Date pit	8	44	48	100
Flaxseed	72	18	10	100
Groundnut	30	50	20	100
Herring	58	27	15	100
Kapok seed	34	46	20	100

* Reprinted with permission from: Spiller, GA. Handbook of Lipids in Human Nutrition. Boca Raton, Florida: CRC Press, Inc., 1996:201-3. Copyright CRC Press, Boca Raton, Florida.

Fatty Acid Content in Selected Fats and Foods *(continued)*

g/100 g

	Polyunsaturated	Monounsaturated	Saturated	Total fat
Lard	11	46	43	100
Linseed	68	21	11	100
Macadamia	4	84	12	100
Mustardseed	32	62	6	100
Murumuru tallow	1	9	90	100
Oat	44	36	20	100
Oiticica	84	6	10	100
Olive	7	83	10	100
Ouri-curi	2	13	85	100
Palm	8	37	55	100
Palm kernel	2	14	84	100
Papaya seed	8	72	20	100
Peanut	32	49	19	100
Perillo	84	8	8	100
Pilchard	59	18	23	100
Poppyseed	62	30	8	100
Rapeseed	23	71	6	100
Rapeseed—low erucic	28	66	6	100
Rice bran	34	46	20	100
Safflower	78	13	9	100
Safflower—high oleic	12	80	8	100
Salmon	51	28	21	100
Sardine	56	22	22	100
Sesame seed	43	42	15	100
Shark liver	44	39	17	100
Shea butter	4	49	47	100
Soybean	59	25	16	100
Sperm—body*	1	86	13	100
Sperm—head*	1	55	44	100
Sunflower seed	70	18	12	100
Tallow—beef	4	43	53	100
Tallow—mutton	5	43	52	100
Teaseed	8	83	9	100
Tucum	3	13	84	100
Tung	79	15	6	100
Ucuhuba tallow	3	7	90	100
Whale	18	55	27	100
Wheat germ	66	18	16	100

---

* Fatty acid averages of glyceride content: 34%—sperm body oil; 26%—sperm head oil. Balance is wax esters.

Fatty Acid Content in Selected Fats and Foods *(continued)*

	g/100 g edible portion		
	Unsaturated	Saturated	Total fat
Raw Whole Foods			
Animal			
Fish			
Catfish	3	1	4
Eel	14	4	18
Herring	13	3	16
Mackerel	9	4	13
Salmon	7	2	9
Trout	8	3	11
Tuna (albacore)	5	3	8
Meats (lean, raw)			
Beef	13	12	25
Mutton	9	6	15
Pork	12	19	31
Rabbit	5	3	8
Venison	1	3	4
Whale	7	1	8
Poultry/eggs			
Chicken w/skin	13	7	20
Chicken—lean	10	4	14
Egg	8	4	12
Turkey w/skin	11	4	15
Turkey—lean	5	2	7
Milk			
Buffalo	4	5	9
Cow	2	2	4
Butter	44	46	81
Goat	2	2	4
Human	2	2	4
Plant			
Cereal and grains			
Maize	3	1	4
Millet	2	1	3
Oats	6	1	7
Rice	1	1	2
Rye	1	1	2
Sorghum	3	1	4
Wheat	1	2	3
Nuts and seeds			
Almond	50	4	54
Beechnut	46	4	50
Brazilnut	54	13	67
Cashew	38	8	46

Fatty Acid Content in Selected Fats and Foods *(continued)*

g/100 g edible portion

	Unsaturated	Saturated	Total fat
Coconut	5	31	36
Filbert	60	5	65
Groundnut	40	10	50
Hickorynut	63	6	69
Peanut	38	10	48
Pecan	45	5	71
Pilinut	38	25	63
Pinenut	49	6	55
Pistachio	49	5	54
Pumpkin	39	8	47
Safflower	55	5	60
Soybean	15	3	18
Sunflower	41	6	47
Walnut	66	7	63

Food and Agriculture Organization of the United Nations, Dietary Fats and Oils in Human Nutrition, report of an expert consultation, Rome, Italy, 1977.

USDA, Composition of Foods: Raw, Processed, Prepared, Agriculture Handbook No. 8, 1963, U.S. Department of Agriculture, Washington, D.C., 1975.

Erasmus, U., Fats and Oils: The Complete Guide to Fats and Oils in Health and Nutrition, Alive Books, Vancouver, B.C., 1986.

Swern, D., Ed., Bailey's Industrial Oil and Fat Products, Vol. 1 and 2, 4th ed., John Wiley & Sons, New York, 1979.

TESTING FOR FATTY ACID STATUS: A LIST OF LABORATORIES

Great Smokies Diagnostic Laboratory
63 Zillicoa St.
Asheville, NC 28801

MetaMetrix Medical Laboratory
5000 Peachtree Ind. Blvd., Suite 110
Norcross, GA 30071

Monro Medical Laboratory
Route 17, P.O. Box 1
Southfield, NY 10975

APPENDIX C

PRACTITIONER REFERRAL

For information about practitioners in your geographic area who are familiar with the concepts of nutrition, functional medicine, or functional laboratory testing you may call 1-800-245-9076. You will be asked to leave your name and address along with your telephone number (in case spelling or other information needs clarification). The names of practitioners in your area will be sent to you at no charge.

ESSENTIAL AND METABOLIC FATTY ACID ANALYSIS (RED BLOOD CELLS)

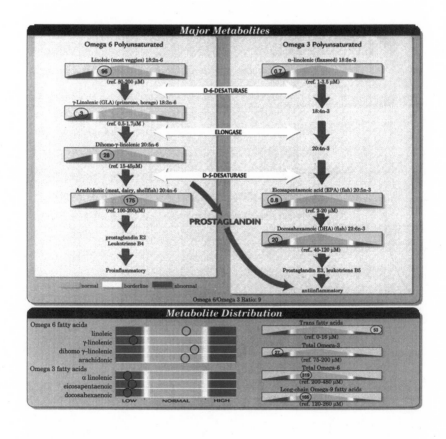

Histograms represent idealized data based upon large populations. Source: Great Smokies Diagnostic Laboratory.

214

REFERENCES

Chapter One

1. Baker, S. Personal communication, 1996.
2. Holman, RT, Johnson, SB, Hatch, TF. A case of human linolenic acid deficiency involving neurological abnormalities. Am J Clin Nutr 1982;35:617–23.
3. Lucas, A, Morley, R, Cole, TJ, et al. Breast milk and subsequent intelligence quotient in children born preterm. Lancet 1992;339: 261–64.
4. Nightingale, S, et al. Red blood cell and adipose tissue fatty acids in active and inactive multiple sclerosis. Acta Neurol Scand 1990;82: 43–50.
5. Adams, P, et al. Arachidonic acid to eicosapentaenoic acid ratio in blood correlates positively with clinical symptoms of depression. Lipids 1996;(Suppl.)31:S-157–61.
6. Stevens, LJ, Burgess, J. Omega-3 fatty acids in boys with behavior, learning, and health problems. Physiology Behavior 1996;59(4–5): 915–20.
7. Virkkunen, ME, Horrobin, DF, Douglas, K, Jenkins, K, Manku, MS. Plasma phospholipid essential fatty acids and prostaglandin in alcoholic, habitually violent, and impulsive offenders. Biol Psych 1987;22:1087–96.
8. Dobbing, J. Vulnerable periods of brain development. In Elliott, K, Knight, E., eds. Lipids Malnutrition and the Developing Brain.

215

Amsterdam: Associated Scientific Publishers, A Ciba Foundation Symposium, Elsevier, 1972:9–22.

9. Sinclair, AJ, Crawford, MA. The effect of a low fat maternal diet on neonatal rats. Br J Nutr 1973;29:127–137.

10. Connor, WE, Neuringer, M. The effects of n-3 fatty acid deficiency and repletion upon the fatty acid composition and function of the brain and retina. In Biological Membranes: Alterations in Membrane Structure and Function. Alan R. Liss Inc., 1988:275–294.

11. Yokota, A. Relationship of polyunsaturated fatty acid composition and learning ability in rat. Nippon Saniujinka Clakkadji (in Japanese)1993;45:15–22.

12. Salem, N, Niebyiski, C. The nervous system has an absolute molecular species requirement for proper function. Mol Memb Biol 1995; 12:131–32.

13. Farquharson, J. Infant cerebral cortex and dietary fatty acids. Eur J Clin Nutr 1994;48(S2):S24–S26.

14. Rudin, DO. Omega-3 essential fatty Acids in medicine. In Bland, JS. 1984–85 Yearbook in Nutritional Medicine, New Canaan, Connecticut: Keats Publishing, Inc., 1985:41.

15. Simopoulos, AP. Omega-3 fatty acids. In Spiller, GA, ed. Handbook of Lipids in Human Nutrition. Boca Raton, Florida: CRC Press, Inc., 1996;51–73.

16. Connor, WE, Neuringer, M, Reisbick, S. Essential fatty acids: The importance of n-3 fatty acids in the retina and brain. Nutr Rev 1992;50(4):21–29.

Chapter Two

1. Bazan, NG. Supply of n-3 polyunsaturated fatty acids and their significance in the central nervous system. In Wurtman, RJ, Wurtman, JJ. eds., Nutrition and the Brain, Vol. 8. New York: Raven Press, Ltd., 1990:2.

2. Glen, AIM, et al. A red cell membrane abnormality in a subgroup of schizophrenic patients: evidence for two diseases. Schiz Res 1994; 12:53–61.

3. Bazan, NG, Gordon, WC, Rodriguez de Turco, EB. The uptake, metabolism and conservation of docosahexaenoic acid (22:6n-3) in brain and retina alterations in liver and retinal 22:6 metabolism during inherited progressive retinal degeneration. In Sinclair, A, Gibson,

R, eds., Essential Fatty Acids and Eicosanoids. Champaign, Illinois: American Oil Chemists' Society, 1992:107–115.

4. Birch, EE, Birch, DG, Hoffman, DR, Uauy, R. Dietary essential fatty acid supply and visual acuity development. Invest Ophthalmol Vis Sci 1992;33(11):3242–53.

5. Simopoulos, AT. Omega-3 fatty acids. In Spiller, GE, ed. Handbook of Lipids in Human Nutrition. Boca Raton, Florida: CRC Press, 1996:58.

6. Bear, MF, Connors, BW, Paradiso, MA. Neuroscience: Exploring the Brain. Baltimore: Williams & Wilkins, 1996:201–206.

7. Baker, S. Environmental Medicine: Comprehensive, Cause Oriented, and Preventive Care. American Academy of Environmental Medicine Symposium, Dearborne, Michigan. 1996.

Chapter Three

1. Galland, L. Personal communication. New York, 1996.

2. Perlmutter, D. Personal communication, Naples, FL, 1996.

3. Bourré, JM. Brainfood. Boston, Massachusetts: Little, Brown and Company, 1993;208–09.

4. Pesonen, E, Hirvonen, J, Karkola, K, et al. Dimensions of the coronary arteries in children. Ann Med 1991;23:85–88.

5. Ibid.

6. Moilanen, T, et al. Tracking of serum fatty acid composition: a 6-year follow-up study in Finnish youths. Am J Epidemiol 1992; 136(12):1487–92.

7. Glueck, CJ, et al. Improvement in symptoms of depression and in an index of life stressor accompany treatment of severe hypertriglyceridemia. Biol Psychiatry 1993;34(4):240–52.

8. Blaun, R. Psychology Today, May/June, 1996:35–43.

9. Ibid.

10. Johnson, H, Russell, JK, Torres, BA. Structural basis for arachidonic acid second messenger signal in gamma-interferon induction. In Biology of the Leukotrienes. Ann NY Acad Sci 1988;524:208–17.

Chapter Four

1. Bourré, JM Francois, M, Youyou, A, et al. The effects of dietary alpha-linolenic acid on the composition of nerve membranes, enzymatic activity, amplitude of electrophysiological parameters, resis-

tance to poisons, and performance of learning tasks in rats. J Nutr 1989;119:1880–92.

2. Simopoulos, AT. Omega-3 fatty acids. In Spiller, GE, ed. Handbook of Lipids in Human Nutrition. Boca Raton, Florida: CRC Press, 1996:68.

3. Innis, S. essential fatty acid requirements in human nutrition. Can J Physiol Pharmacol 1993;71(1):699–706.

4. Innis, S, Nelson, C, Rioux, M, King, D. Development of visual acuity in relation to plasma and erythrocyte omega-6 and omega-3 fatty acids in healthy term gestation infants. Am J Clin Ntur 1994;60(3): 347–52.

5. Rudin, DO, Felix, C. The Omega-3 Phenomenon. New York: Rawson Associates, 1987.

6. Rudin, DO. Modernization disease syndrome as substrate pellagra-beriberi. J Orthomolecular Med 1987;2(1):3–14.

7. Ibid.

8. Farquharson, J, Jamieson, EC, Abbasi, KA, Patrick, WJA, Logan, RW, Cockburn, F. Effect of diet on the fatty acid composition of the major phospholipids of infant cerebral cortex. Arch Dis Child 1995; 72:198–203.

9. Ibid.

10. Stubbs, CD. The structure and function of docosahexaenoic acid in membranes. In Sinclair, A, Gibson, R, eds., Essential Fatty Acids and Eicosanoids. Champaign, Illinois: American Oil Chemists' Society, 1992:116.

11. Farquharson, J. Infant cerebral cortex and dietary fatty acids. Eur J Clin Nutr 1994;48 (S-2):S24–S26.

12. Carlson, SE, Werkman, SH, Rhodes, PG, Tolley, EA. Visual acuity development in healthy preterm infants: effect of marine-oil supplementation. Am J Clin Nutr 1993;58:35–42.

13. Lucas, A, Morley, R, Cole, TJ, et al. Breast milk and subsequent intelligence quotient in children born preterm. Lancet 1992;339:261.

14. Bazan, N. Supply of n-3 polyunsaturated fatty acids and their significance in the central nervous system. In Wurtman, RJ, Wurtman, JJ, eds. Nutrition and the Brain, Vol. 8. New York: Raven Press, Ltd. 1990:1–22.

15. Kinko, Y-Y, Hayakawa, K. Docosahexaenoic acid: A valuable nutraceutical? Trends Food Sci Tech 1996:Feb; 59–63.

16. Ibid.

17. Ibid.

18. Agren, JJ, et al. Fatty acid composition of erythrocyte, platelet, and serum lipids in strict vegetarians. Lipids 1995;30(4):365–69.
19. Reddy, S, Sanders, TAB, Obeid, O. The influence of maternal vegetarian diet on essential fatty acid status of the newborn. Eur J Clin Nutr 1994;48:358–68.
20. Sanders, TAB, Reddy, S. The influence of a vegetarian diet on the fatty acid composition of milk and the essential fatty acid status of the infant. J Pediatr 1992;120:S71–77.
21. Passwater, R. Evening primrose oil. In Barilla, J. ed., The Nutrition Superbook: The Good Fats and Oils. New Canaan, Connecticut: Keats Publishing, Inc., 1995:91–92.
22. Galland, L. Personal communication. New York, 1996.
23. Passwater, R. Evening primrose oil. In Barilla, J. ed., The Nutrition Superbook: The Good Fats and Oils. New Canaan, Connecticut: Keats Publishing, Inc., 1995:91–92.
24. Kimura, D, Hampson, E. Neural and hormonal mechanisms mediating sex differences in cognition. Research Bulletin No. 689. London, Ontario: Department of Psychology, University of Western Ontario, 1990.
25. Golier, JA, et al. Low serum cholesterol and attempted suicide. Am J Psychiatry 1995;152:419–23.
26. Tankins, T. Study questions harmful effect of cholesterol in eggs. Med Trib 1995;March.
27. Put, A, et al. Clinical efficacy of 'essential' phospholipids in patients chronically exposed to organic solvents. J Intl Med Res 1993;21:185–91.
28. Hirata, F, Axelrod, J. Phospholipid methylation and biological signal transmission. Science 1980;209:1082–90.
29. Amaducci, L, Crook, TH, Lippi, A, et al. Use of phosphatidylserine in Alzheimer's Disease. Ann NY Acad Sci 1991;640:245–49.
30. Woodbury, MM, Woodbury, MA. Neuropsychiatric development: Two case reports about the use of dietary fish oils and/or choline supplementation in children. J Am Col Nutr 1993;12(3):239–45.
31. Kidd, P. Phosphatidylserine: A Remarkable Brain Cell Nutrient. Decatur, Illinois: Lucas Meyer, 1995:2.

Chapter Five

1. Siguel, EN, Lerman, RH. Prevalence of essential fatty acid deficiency in patients with chronic gastrointestinal disorders. Metabolism 1996;45:12–23.
2. Sokol, RJ. Vitamin E deficiency and neurologic disease. Ann Rev Nutr 1988;8:351–73.
3. Lugea, A, Videla, S, Vilaseca, J, Guarner, F. Antiulcerogenic and anti-inflammatory action of fatty acids on the gastrointestinal tract. Prost Leuk Ess Fat Acids 1991;43:135–140.
4. Wester, P. Magnesium. Am J Clin Nutr 1987;45:1305–12.
5. Franz, KB. Magnesium intake during pregnancy. Magnesium 1987; 6:18–27.
6. Rea, W. Chemical Sensitivity. Boca Raton, Florida: Lewis Publishers, 1993:256.
7. Holden, JM, et al. Zinc and copper in self-selected diets. J Am Diet Assoc 1979;75:23.
8. Kant, AK, Block, G. Dietary vitamin B6 intake and food sources in the US population: NHANES II, 1976–1980. Am J Clin Nutr 1990; 52:707–16.
9. Heller, S. Vitamin B6 status in pregnancy. Am J Clin Nutr 1973; 26(12):1339–48.
10. Horrobin, DF. Gamma-linolenic acid in medicine. In Bland, JS. 1984–85 Yearbook of Nutritional Medicine. New Canaan, Connecticut: Keats Publishing, Inc., 1985;25–26.
11. Pawlosky, RJ, Salem, N. Ethanol exposure causes a decrease in docosahexaenoic acid and an increase in docosapentaenoic acid in feline brains and retinas. Am J Clin Nutr 1995;61:1284–89.
12. Salem, N. Alcohol, fatty acids, and diet. Alc Hlth Res Wrld 1898; 13(3):211–18.
13. Bland, JS. The 20–day Rejuvenation Diet Program. New Canaan, Connecticut: Keats Publishing, Inc. 1996:71.
14. Foster-Powell, K, Miller, JB. International tables of glycemic index. Am J Clin Nutr 1995;62:871S-93S.

Chapter Six

1. Halliwell, B, Gutteridge, JMC. Free Radicals in Biology and Medicine. 2nd ed. New York: Oxford University Press, 1989:264–65.
2. Ibid.

3. Bourré, JM. Brainfood. Boston: Little, Brown and Company, 1993; 56. Bourre reports on the work of neuroscientist Nicholas Bazan.
4. Benzi, G, Moretti, A. Age and peroxidative stress-related modifications of the cerebral enzymatic activities linked to mitochondria and the glutathione system. Free Rad Biol Med 1995;19(1):77–101.
5. Beal, F. Mitochondria in neurodegenerative disease. Third International Symposium on Functional Medicine, Vancouver, British Columbia, 1996.
6. Travis, J. Do brain cells run out of gas? Science News 1995;148(6): 84–85.
7. McGuire, JJ, et al. Succinate-ubiquinone reductase linked to recycling of alpha-tocopherol in reconstituted systems and mitochondria: requirement for reduced ubiquinol. Arch Biochem Biophys 1992;292:47–53.
8. Kristal, B, Park, BJ, Yu, BP. Antioxidants reduce peroxyl-mediated inhibition of mitochondrial transcription. Free Rad Biol Med 1994; 16(5):653–60.
9. Kehrer, JP, Lund, LG. Cellular reducing equivalents and oxidative stress. Free Rad Biol Med 1994;17(1):65–75.
10. Shoffner, JM, Wallace, DC. Oxidative phosphorylation disease and mitochondrial DNA mutations: Diagnosis and treatment. Annu Rev Nutr 1994;14:353–68.
11. Leibovitz, B, Mueller, J. Bioflavonoids and polyphenols: medical applications. J Opt Nutr 1993;2(1):17–35.
12. Packer, L, Witt, E, Tritschler, H. Alpha-lipoic acid as a biological antioxidant. Free Rad Biol Med 1995;19(2):227–50.
13. Reed, DJ. Oxidative stress and mitochondrial permeability transition. In Packer, L, Cadenas, E, eds., Biothiols in Health and Disease. New York: Marcel Dekker, Inc., 1995:231–63.
14. Miyazawa, T. Membrane phospholipid hydroperoxides as estimated by chemiluminescence: The effect of dietary polyunsaturated fatty acids. In Sinclair, A, Gibson, A, eds., Essential Fatty Acids and Eicosanoids. Champaign, Illinois: American Oil Chemists Society, 1992:383–88.
15. Fahn, S. A pilot trial of high-dose alpha-tocopherol and ascorbate in early Parkinson's disease. Ann Neurol 1992;32(Supple):S128–S132.
16. Ziegler, D, Gries, FA, Therapeutic effects of alpha-lipoic acid on diabetic neuropathy. In Packer, L, Cadenas, E, eds., Biothiols in Heatlh and Disease. New York, NY: Marcel Dekker, Inc. 1995: 467–77.

17. Bakker, HD, Scholte, HR, Jeneson, JA. Vitamin E in a mitochondrial myopathy with proliferating mitochondria. Lancet 1993;342 (8864):1175–76.
18. Sokol, RJ. Vitamin E deficiency and neurologic disease. Ann Rev Nutr 1988;8:351–73.
19. Laganiere, S, Fernandes, G. High peroxidizability of subcellular membrane induced by high fish oil diet is reversed by vitamin E. Clin Res 1987;35(3):565A.
20. Bland, JS, Benum, S. The 21–day Rejuvenation Diet Program. New Canaan, Connecticut: Keats Publishing, Inc. 1996:102–03.
21. Antioxidant content of vegetables, teas measured. Food Chemical News 1996;12:9.

Chapter Seven

1. Lees, RS, Lees, RS, Karel, M, eds., Impact of dietary fat on human health. In Omega-3 Fatty Acids in Health and Disease. New York: Marcel Dekker, 1990:1.
2. Dopeshwarkar, GA. Nutrition and Brain Development. New York: Plenum Press, 1981:70–73.
3. Grandgirard, A, Bourré, JM, Julliard, F, et al. Incorporation of trans long-chain n-3 polyunsaturated fatty acids in rat brain structure and retina. Lipids 1994;29(4):251–58.
4. Petersen, J, Opstvedt, J. Trans fatty acids: Fatty acid composition of lipids of the brain and other organs in suckling piglets. Lipids 1992; 27(10):761–69.
5. de Schrjver, R, Privett, OS. Interrelationship between dietary trans fatty acids and the 6- and 9- desaturases in the rat. Lipids 1982; 17:27.
6. Mahfouz, MM, Smith, TL, Kummerow, FA. Effect of dietary fats on desaturase activities and the biosynthesis of fatty acids in rat-liver microsomes. 1984;19:214.
7. Dopeshwarkar, GA. Nutrition and Brain Development. New York: Plenum Press, 1981:70–73.
8. Holman, RT, Pusch, F, Svingen, B, Dutton, HJ. Unusual isomeric polyunsaturated fatty acids in liver phospholipids of rats fed hydrogenated oil. Proc Natl Acad Sci USA 1991;88:4830.
9. Simopoulos, AT. Trans Fatty Acids. In Spiller, GE, ed. Handbook of Lipids in Human Nutrition. Boca Raton, Florida: CRC Press, 1996: 96.

10. Enig, MG, Subodh, A, Keeney, M, Sampugna, J. Isomeric trans fatty acids in the U.S. diet. J Am Col Nutr 1990;9(5):471–86.
11. Desci, T, Thiel, I, Koletzko, B. Essential fatty acids in full term infants fed breast milk or formula. Arch Dis Child 1995;72:F23–F28.
12. Chen, ZY, Pelletier, G, Hollywood, R, Ratnayake, WMN. Trans fatty acid isomers in Canadian human milk. Lipids 1995;30(1): 15–21.
13. Ibid.
14. Crawford, M, Marsh, D. Nutrition and Evolution. New Canaan, Connecticut: Keats Publishing, 1995:185.
15. van den Reek, M, Craig-Schmidt, M, Weete, J, et al. Fat in the diets of adolescent girls with emphasis on isomeric fatty acids. Am J Clin Nutr 1986;Apr. 3;530–37.
16. Simopoulos, AT. Trans fatty acids. In Spiller, GE, ed. Handbook of Lipids in Human Nutrition. Boca Raton, Florida: CRC Press, 1996: 96.

Chapter Eight

1. Roohr-Hyzer, GJ. Personal communication, 1996.
2. Connor, WE, Neuringer, M, Reisbick, S.. Essential fatty acids: The importance of n-3 fatty acids in the retina and brain. Nutr Rev 1992;50(4):21–29.
3. Van Jaarsveld, PJ, et al. The essential fatty acid status of women from a community with low socioeconomic status. Med Sci Res 1994;22:719–21.
4. Holman, RT, Johnson, SB, Ogburn, PL. Deficiency of essential fatty acids and membrane fluidity during pregnancy and lactation. Proc Nat Acad Sci 1991;88:4835–4839.
5. Ibid.
6. Al, MDM, van Houwelingen, AC, Hornstra, G. The effect of pregnancy on the cervonic acid (docosahexaenoic acid) status of mothers and their newborns. Department of Human Biology, University of Limburg, Maastricht, The Netherlands. Second Internationl Congress of International Society for Study of Fatty Acids and Lipids. Washington, D.C., June 8–11, 1995.
7. Holman, RT, Johnson, SB, Ogburn, PL. Deficiency of essential fatty acids and membrane fluidity during pregnancy and lactation. Proc Nat Acad Sci 1991;88:4835–4839.

8. Crawford, M. The role of essential fatty acids in neural development: implications for perinatal nutrition. Am J Clin Nutr 1993; 57(suppl.):703S-710S.

9. Kane, P. Personal communication, Reno, Nevada, 1996.

10. Farquharson, J, Jamieson, EC, Abbasi, KA, Patrick, WJA, Logan, RW, Cockburn, F. Effect of diet on the fatty acid composition of the major phospholipids of infant cerebral cortex. Arch Dis Child 1995;72:198–203.

11. Innis, S. Essential fatty acid requirements in human nutrition. Can J Physiol Pharmacol 1993;71(1):699–706.

12. Innis, S, Nelson, C, Rioux, M, King, D. Development of visual acuity in relation to plasma and erythrocyte omega-6 and omega-3 fatty acids in healthy term gestation infants. Am J Clin Ntur 1994; 60(3):347–52.

13. Lucas, A, Morley, R, Cole, TJ, et al. Breast milk and subsequent intelligence quotient in children born preterm. Lancet 1992;339:261.

14. Simopoulos, AT. Omega-3 Fatty Acids. In Spiller, GE, ed. Handbook of Lipids in Human Nutrition. Boca Raton, Florida: CRC Press, 1996:68.

15. Innis, S. Essential fatty acid requirements in human nutrition. Can J Physiol Pharmacol 1993;71(1):699–706.

16. Ibid.

17. Anonymous. Organochlorines lace Inuit breast milk. Sci News 1994;Feb 12;111.

18. Gibson, R. What is the best fatty acid composition for the fats of infant formula? In Sinclair, A, Gibson, R, eds. Essential Fatty Acids and Eicosanoids. Champaign, Illinois: American Oil Chemists' Society, 1992:210–13.

19. Farquharson, J. Infant cerebral cortex and dietary fatty acids. Eur J Clin Nutr 1994;48(S2):S24–S26.

20. Farquharson, J, Jamieson, EC, Abbasi, KA, Patrick, WJA, Logan, RW, Cockburn, F. Effect of diet on the fatty acid composition of the major phospholipids of infant cerebral cortex. Arch Dis Child 1995; 72:198–203.

21. Kennedy, E, Goldberg, J. What are American children eating?: Implications for public policy. Nutr Rev 1995;53(5):111–26.

22. St. Jeor, S. The role of weight management in the health of women. J Am Diet Assoc 1993;9.

23. Rodin, J. Body Traps. New York: Quill William Morrow Press, 1992;34.

24. Pawlosky, RJ, Salem, N. Ethanol exposure causes a decrease in docosahexaenoic acid and an increase in docosapentaenoic acid in feline brains and retinas. Am J Clin Nutr 1995;61:1284–89.
25. Kyle, D. Communication of unpublished observations, 1997.
26. Markesbury, P. Communication of unpublished observations, 1997.
27. Rickkinen, P. Communication of unpublished observations, 1997.
28. Schaefer, E. Decreased plasma phosphatidylcholine docosahexaenoic acid content in dementia. Keeping Your Brain in Shape, Roundtable Discussion. Cornell University School of Medicine, April 1997.

Chapter Nine

1. Crayhon, R. Personal communication, New York, 1995.
2. Hibbeln, JR, Salem, N. Dietary polyunsaturated fatty acids and depression: when cholesterol does not satisfy. Am J Clin Nutr 1995; 62:1–9.
3. Ibid.
4. Ibid.
5. Cross National Collaborative Group. The changing rate of major depression across national comparisons. JAMA 1992;268:3098–105.
6. Chen, C, Wong, J, Lee, N, et al. The Shatin community mental health survey in Hong Kong II. Major findings. Arch Gen Psychiatry 1993;50:125–33.
7. Hirayasu, A. An epidemiological and sociopsychiatric study on the mental and neurologic disorders in an isolated island in Okinawa. Psychiatry Neurol Jpn 1969;71:466–91.
8. Hasegawa, K. The epidemiological study of depression in later life. J Affect Disord 1985;S1:S3–6.
9. Burton, R. The Anatomy of Melancholy. The Classics of Psychiatry and Behavioral Sciences Library. Birmingham, Alabama: Division of Gryphon Editions, Inc., 1988.
10. Adams, P, et al. Arachidonic acid to eicosapentaenoic acid ratio in blood correlates positively with clinical symptoms of depression. Lipids 1996;(Suppl.)31:S-157–61.
11. Maes, M. Fatty acid composition in major depression: decreased n-3 fractions in cholesteryl esters and increased C20:4n-6/C20:5n-3 ratio in cholesteryl esters and phospholipids. J Affect Dis 1996;38: 35–46.

12. Blaun, R. Psychology Today, May/June, 1996;35–43.

13. Glueck, CJ, et al. Improvement in symptoms of depression and in an index of life stressor accompany treatment of severe hypertriglyceridemia. Biol Psychiatry 1993;34(4):240–52.

14. Simopoulos, AP. Omega-3 fatty acids. In Spiller, GA, ed. Handbook of Lipids in Human Nutrition. Boca Raton, Florida: CRC Press, Inc., 1996;51–73.

15. Al, MDM, van Houwelingen, AC, Hornstra, G. The effect of pregnancy on the cervonic acid (docosahexaenoic acid) status of mothers and their newborns. Department of Human Biology, University of Limburg, Maastricht, The Netherlands. Second International Congress of International Society for Study of Fatty Acids and Lipids. Washington, D.C., June 8–11, 1995.

16. Hibbeln, J, Salem, N. Dietary polyunsaturated fatty acids and depression: when cholesterol does not satisfy. Am J Clin Nutr 1995; 62:1–9.

17. Neziroglu, F, Nemone, R, Yaryura-Tobias, JA. Onset of obsessive-compulsive disorder in pregnancy. Am J Psychiatry 1992;149:947–50.

18. Schubert, DSP, Foliart, RH. Increased depression in multiple sclerosis patients: a meta-analysis. Psychosomatics 1993;34:124–30.

19. Nightingale, S, Woo, E, Smith, AD, et al. Red blood cell and adipose tissue fatty acids in active and inactive multiple sclerosis. Acta Neurol Scand 1990;82:43–50.

20. Holman, RT, Johnson, SB, Ogburn, PL. Deficiency of essential fatty acids and membrane fluidity during pregnancy and lactation. Proc Nat Acad Sci 1991;88:4835–39.

21. Sengupta, N, Datta, SC, Sengupta, D. Platelet and erythrocyte membrane lipid and phospholipid patterns in different types of mental patients. Biochem Med 1981;25:267–75.

22. Gindin, J, et al. The effect of plant phosphatidylserine on age-associated memory impairment and mood in the functioning elderly. Geriatric Inst for Ed Res, and Department of Geriatrics, Kaplan Hospital, Rhovot, Israel, 1995.

23. Ibid.

24. Maggioni, M, et al. Effects of phosphatidylserine therapy in geriatric subjects with depressive disorders. Acta Psychiatr Scand 1990;81:265–70.)(Manfredi, M, et al. Risultati clinici della fosfatidil-serina in 40 donne affette da turb psico-organiche, in eta clima-

terica e senile. La Clinica Terapeutica 1987;120:33–36 [English summary].

25. Behan, PO, Behan, WMH, Horrobin, DF. Placebo-controlled trial of n-3 and n-6 essential fatty acids in the treatment of post-viral fatigue syndrome. Acta Neurologica Scandinavica 1990;82:209–16.

26. Mitchell, EA, Aman, MG, Turbott, SH, Manku, M. Clinical characteristics and serum essential fatty acid levels in hyperactive children. Clin Pediatr 1987;26:406–11.

27. Burgess, JR, et al. Essential fatty acid metabolism in boys with attention deficit-hyperactivity disorder. A J Clin Nutr 1995;62:761–68.

28. Stevens, LJ, et al. Omega-3 fatty acids in boys with behavior, learning, and health problems. Physiology Behavior 1996;59(4–5):915–20.

29. Baker, S. Personal communication, 1996.

30. Kaplan, JR, Manuk, SB, Shively, C. The effects of fat and cholesterol on social behavior in monkeys. Psychosom Med 1991;53:634–642.

31. Muldoon, MF, et al. Effects of a low-fat diet on brain serotonergic responsivity in cynomolgus monkeys. Biol Psychiatry 1992;31:739–42.

32. Kaplan, JR, et al. Cholesterol restriction alters central serotonergic activity and social behavior in monkeys. Am J Primatol (in press).

33. Fiennes, RN, Sinclair, AJ, Crawford, MA. Essential fatty acid studies in primates: Linolenic acid requirements of Capuchins. J Med Primat 1973;2:155–69.)

34. Virkkunen, ME, Horrobin, DF, Douglas, K, Jenkins, K, Manku, MS. Plasma phospholipid essential fatty acids and prostaglandins in alcoholic, habitually violent, and impulsive offenders. Biol Psych 1987;22:1087–96.

35. Pawlosky, RJ, Salem, N. Ethanol exposure causes a decrease in docosahexaenoic acid and an increase in docosapentaenoic acid in feline brains and retinas. Am J Clin Nutr 1995;61:1284–89.

36. Christiansen, O, Christiansen, E. Fat consumption and schizophrenia. Acta Psychiatr Scand 1988;78:587–91.

37. Glen, AIM, et al. A red cell membrane abnormality in a subgroup of schizophrenic patients: Evidence for two diseases. Schiz Res 1994; 12:53–61.

38. Laugharne, JDE, et al. Fatty acids and schizophrenia. Lipids 1996; 31(S):S-163–65.

39. Peet, M. Essential fatty acid deficiency in erythrocyte membranes from chronic schizophrenic patients and the clinical effects of dietary supplementation. Prost Leukotr Ess Fat Acids 1996;55(1&2): 71–75.

40. Passwater, R. Evening primrose oil. In Barilla, J. ed. The Nutrition Superbook: The Good Fats and Oils. New Canaan, Connecticut: Keats Publishing, Inc., 1995:96.

41. Sosnovskii, AS, et al. Activity of antioxidant enzymes in the limbic reticular structures of rat brain after short-term immobilization. Byull Eksp Biol Med 1993;115;683–85.

42. Sosnovskii, AS, et al. Lipid peroxidation in rats with emotional stress: correlation with open field behavior. Byull Eksp Biol Meditsin 1992;113:19–21.

43. Avdulov, NA, et al. Changes in synaptosomal membranes from cerebral cortex due to psychogenic stress in rats. Ann 1st Super Sanita 1990;26:31–6.

44. Bear, MF, Connors, BW, Paradiso, MA. Neuroscience: Exploring the Brain. Baltimore: Williams & Wilkins, 1996:412.

45. Mills, DE, Prkachin, KM, Harvey, KA, Ward, RP. Dietary fatty acid supplementation alters stress reactivity and performance in man. J Human Hypertension 1989;3:111–16.

46. Monteleone, P, Beinat, L, Tanzillo, C, et al. Effects of phosphatidylserine on the neuroendocrine response to physical stress in humans. Neuroendocrinology 1990;52:243–48.

47. Monteleone, P. Blunting by chronic phosphatidylserine administration of the stress-induced activation of the hypothalamo-pituitary-adrenal axis in healthy men. Eur J Clin Pharmacol (Germany) 1992; 42:385–88.

48. Hibbeln, JR, Salem, N. Dietary polyunsaturated fatty acids and depression: When cholesterol does not satisfy. Am J Clin Nutr 1995; 62:1–9.

Chapter Ten

1. Shapiro, V. Personal communication, Duluth, Minnesota, 1996.
2. Ibid.
3. Swank, R, Dugan, BB. The Multiple Sclerosis Diet Book. Garden City, New York: Doubleday & Co., Inc., 1987.

4. Nightingale, S, Woo, E, Smith, AD, et al. Red blood cell and adipose tissue fatty acids in active and inactive multiple sclerosis. Acta Neurol Scand 1990;82:43–50.

5. Piscane, A, et al. Breast feeding and multiple sclerosis. Br Med J 1994;308:1411–12.

6. Gusev, Y. Russian State Medical University. Personal communication, 1996.

7. Claussen, J, Moller, J. Allergic encephalomyelitis induced by brain antigen after deficiency in polyunsaturated fatty acids during myelination. Acta Neurol Scand 1967;43:375–88.

8. Sibley, WA. Therapeutic claims committee of the International Federation of Multiple Sclerosis Societies. Therapeutic Claims in Multiple Sclerosis. New York: Demos Publications, 1992.

9. Bates, D. Dietary lipids and multiple sclerosis. Uppsala J Med Sci 1990(Suppl);48:1973–87.

10. Wozniak-Wowk, CS. Nutrition intervention in the management of multiple sclerosis. Nutr Today 1993;25(6):12–22.

11. Ibid.

12. Perlmutter, D. Personal communication. Naples, Florida, 1996.

13. Fatty acid reportedly lowers stroke. Med Trib 1995;June 8:20.

14. Gillman, MW, et al. A protective effect of fruits and vegetables on development of stroke in men. JAMA 1995;273(14):1113–17.

15. Jamrozik, K, Broadhurst, RJ, Anderson, CS, Stewart-Wynne, EG. The role of lifestyle factors in the etiology of stroke: A population-based case-control study in Perth, Western Australia. Stroke 1994;25:51–59.

16. Gerster, H. n-3 fish oil polyunsaturated fatty acids and bleeding.1995;281–96.

17. Pauletto, P, et al. Blood pressure, serum lipids, and fatty acids in populations on a lake-fish diet or on a vegetarian diet in Tanzania. Lipids 1996;(Suppl)(31):S309–12.

18. Pauletto, P. Blood pressure and atherogenic lipoprotein profiles of fish-diet and vegetarian villagers in Tanzania: The Lugalawa study. Lancet 1996;348:784–88.

19. Faruque, O, et al. Relationship between smoking and antioxidant nutrient status. Br J Nutr 1995;73:625–32.

20. McLennan, PL, Abeywardena, MY, Charnock, JS. Influence of dietary lipids on arrhythmias and infarction after coronary artery ligation in rats. Can J Physiol Pharmacol 1985;63:1411–17.

21. Kang, JX, Leaf, A. The cardiac antiarrhythmic effects of polyunsaturated fatty acid. Lipids 1996;31:S41–S44.
22. Glueck, CJ. Amelioration of severe migraine with omega-3 fatty acids: a double-blind, placebo-controlled clinical trial. Am J Clin Nutr 1986;43:710.
23. McCarren, T. Amelioration of severe migraine by fish oil (n-3) fatty acids. Am J Clin Nutr 1985;41:874a.
24. Martin, DD, Robbins, MEC, Spector, AA, Chen Wen, B, Hussey, DH. The fatty acid composition of human gliomas differs from that found in nonmalignant brain tissue. Lipds 1996;31(12):1283–88.
25. Ledwozyw, A, Lutnicki, K. Phospholipids and fatty acids in human brain tumors. Acta Physiol Hungarica 1992;79:381–87.
26. White, HB. Normal and neoplastic human brain tissues: Phospholipid, fatty acid and unsaturation number modifications in tumors. In Wood, R, ed. Tumor Lipids: Biochemistry and Metabolism. Champaign, Illinois: American Oil Chemists' Society, 1973:75–88.
27. Martin, DD, Robbins, MEC, Spector, AA, Chen Wen, B, Hussey, DH. The fatty acid composition of human gliomas differs from that found in nonmalignant brain tissue. Lipids 1996;31(12):1283–88.
28. Baker, S. Fatty acids, membranes, and prostaglandins. In Nutrition as it Relates to Environmental Medicine. Part IV: Environmental Medicine: Comprehensive, Cause Oriented Preventive Care. Dearborne, Michigan, 1996:336–41.
29. Spirer, Z, Koren, L, Finkelstein, A, Jurgenson, U. Prevention of febrile seizures by dietary supplementation with n-3 polyunsaturated fatty acids. Med Hyp 1994;43:43–45.
30. Hoffman, DR, Birch, DG. Docosahexaenoic acid in red blood cells of patients with X-linked retinitis pigmentosa. Invest Ophthalmol Vis Sci 1995;36(6):1009–18.
31. Bazan, NG, Scott, BL, Reddy, TS, Pelias, MZ. Decreased content of docosahexanoate and arachidonate in plasma phospholipids in Usher's syndrome. Biochem Biophys Res Comm 1986;141(2):600–04.
32. Werbach, MR. Diabetic neuropathies. Towns Let Doc 1996:22.
33. Keen, H, Payan, J, et al. Treatment of diabetic neuropathy with gamma-linolenic acid. Diabetes Care 1993;16(1):8–15.
34. Werbach, MR. Diabetic neuropathies. Towns Let Doc 1996:22.
35. Bland, J. Functional Medicine Update. Gig Harbor, Washington: Healthcomm, Intl. January, 1997. (Horrobin's work is reviewed.)

36. Bourré, JM, Youyou, A, Durand, G, Pascal, G. Slow recovery of the fatty acid composition of sciatic nerve in rats fed a diet intially low in n-3 fatty acids. Lipids 1987;22(7):535–38.

37. Holman, RT, Johnson, SB, Hatch, TF. A case of human linolenic acid deficiency involving neurological abnormalities. Am J Clin Nutr 1982;35:617–23.

38. Leaf, AA, Leighfield, MJ, Casteloe, KL, Crawford, MA. Factors affecting long-chain polyunsaturated fatty acid composition of plasma choline phosphoglycerides in preterm infants. J Pediatr Gastroenterol Nutr 1992 (in press).

39. Carlson, SE, Rhodes, PG, Ferguson, MG. Docosahexaenoic acid status of preterm infants at birth and following feeding with human milk formula. AM J Clin Nutr 1986;44:798–04.

40. Schaefer, EJ. Decreased plasma phosphatidylcholine docosahexaenoic acid content in dementia. Presented at: Keeping Your Brain in Shape: New Insights into DHA. Cornell University Medical Center, New York, New York, April 8, 1997.

41. Yazawa, K. Clinical experience with docosahexaenoic acid in demented patients. International Conference on Highly Unsaturated Fatty Acids in Nutrition and Disease Prevention, Barcelona, Spain, 1996;November 4–6.

42. Corrigan, FM, Van Rhijn, A, Horrobin, DF. Essential fatty acids in Alzheimer's disease. Ann NY Acad Sci 1991;640:250–2.

43. Brooksbank, BWL, Martinez, M. Lipid abnormalities in the brain in adult Down syndrome and Alzheimer's disease. In Horrocks, LA, ed. Molecular and Chemical Neuropathathology. Humana Press, Inc: London, 1989:157–85.

44. Frolich, L, et al. Free radical mechanisms in dementia of Alzheimer's type and potential for antioxidative treatment. Drug Rsrch 1995; 45(1):443–46.

45. Crook, T, Petrie, W, Wells, C, Massari, DC. Effects of phosphatidlyserine in Alzheimer's disease. Psychopharmacol Bull 1992;28:61–66.

46. Salvioli, G, Neri, M, et al. L-Acetylcarnitine treatment on mental decline in the elderly. Drug Exp Clin Res 1994;20(4):169–76.

47. Woodbury, MM, Woodbury, MA. Neuropsychiatric development: Two case reports about the use of dietary fish oils and/or choline supplementation in children. J Am Col Nutr 1993;12(3):239–45.

48. Brooksbank, BWL, Martinez, M. Lipid abnormalities in the brain in adult Down syndrome and Alzheimer's disease. In Horrocks, LA,

ed. Molecular and Chemical Neuropathathology. Humana Press, Inc: London, 1989:157–85.

49. Thomas, C. Oxidative Stress and Degenerative Disease in Downs. San Diego, California: Pantox Laboratories, 1995. Unpublished mongraph.

50. Bralley, JA. Personal communication, Norcross, Georgia, 1995.

51. Rudin, DO. The major psychoses and neuroses as omega-3 essential fatty acid deficiency syndrome: Substrate pellagra. Biol Phsychiat 1981;16(9):837.

Chapter Eleven

1. Hawking, S. A Brief History of Time. New York: Bantam Books, 1988.

2. Goleman, D. Emotional Intelligence. New York: Bantam, 1995:33.

3. "Warning by a Valedictorian Who Faced Prison." New York Times 1992;June 23.

4. Gardner, H. Frames of Mind: The Theory of Multiple Intelligences. New York: Basic Books, 1983.

5. Buzan, A. Buzan's Book of Genius.

6. Goleman, D. Emotional Intelligence. New York: Bantam, 1995.

7. Schmidt, J. Personal communication regarding presentation at Rudolph Steiner College, Fair Oaks, California, 1995.

8. Yokota, A. Relationship of polyunsaturated fatty acid composition and learning ability in rat. Nippon Saniujinka Clakkadji (in Japanese)1993:45;15–22.

9. Blaun, R. Brain Food: How to eat smart. Psychology Today, May/June 1996;38. Prepublication results of C.E. Greenwood et al are cited.

10. Liu, X, et al. The effects of omega-3 fish oil enriched with DHA on memory. Fatty Acids and Lipids from Cell Biology to Human Disease: 2nd International Congress of the ISSFAL International Society for the Study of Fatty Acids and Lipids; June 7–10, 1995: Congress Programs and Abstracts.

11. Lucas, A, Morley, R, Cole, TJ, et al. Breast milk and subsequent intelligence quotient in children born preterm. Lancet 1992;339:261.

12. Stevens, LJ, et al. Omega-3 fatty acids in boys with behavior, learning, and health problems. Physiology Behavior 1996;59(4–5):915–20.

13. Siguel, E. Essential Fatty Acids in Health and Disease. Brookline, Massachusetts: Nutrek Press, 1994:47.

14. Stordy, BJ. Benefit of docosahexaenoic acid supplements to dark adaption in dyslexics. Lancet 1995;346:385.

15. Kane, P. Personal communication, New Jersey, 1996.

16. Kidd, P. Phosphatidylserine: A Remarkable Brain Cell Nutrient. Decatur, Illinois: Lucas Meyer, Inc. 1995.

17. Crook, TH, et al. Effect of phosphatidylserine in age-associated memory impairment. Neurol 1991;41:644–49.

18. Crook, TH, et al. Effect of phosphatidylserine in Alzheimer's disease. Psychopharmacol Bull 1992;28:61–66.

19. Nunzi, MG, et al. Dendritic spine loss in hippocampus of aged rats: Effect of brain phosphatidylserine administration. Neurobiology Aging 1987;8:501–510.

20. Nunzi, MG, et al. Therapeutic properties of phosphatidylserine in the aging brain. In Hanin, I, Pepeu, G, eds. Phospholipids: Biochemical, Pharmaceutical, and Analytical Considerations. New York: Plenum Press, 1990.

21. Wurtman, RJ, Zeisel, SH. Brain choline: its sources and effects on the synthesis and release of acetylcholine. Aging 1982;19:303–313.

22. Boyd, WE, McQueen, J. Lancet 1977;2:711.

23. Wozniak-Wowk, CS. Nutrition intervention in the management of multiple sclerosis. Nutr Today 1993;25(6):12–22.

24. Galland, L. Personal communication. 1996.

25. Perlmutter, D. Personal communication. 1996.

26. Block, J. Unpublished manuscript. University of California at Berkeley. 1995. Block describes his concept of "ego resilience." It is reviewed in Goleman's Emotional Intelligence.

27. Hibbeln, JR, Salem, N. Dietary polyunsaturated fatty acids and depression: When cholesterol does not satisfy. Am J Clin Nutr 1995; 62:1–9.

28. Burgess, JR, et al. Essential fatty acid metabolism in boys with attention deficit-hyperactivity disorder. A J Clin Nutr 1995;62:761–8.

29. Stevens, LJ, et al. Omega-3 fatty acids in boys with behavior, learning, and health problems. Physiology Behavior 1996;59(4–5):915–20.

30. Galland, L. Personal communication. 1996.

31. Baker, S. Personal communication. 1996.

32. Hamazaki, T, et al. The effect of docosahexaenoic acid on aggression in young adults. J Clin Invest 1996;97:1129–34.

33. Hibbeln, JR, Salem, N. Dietary polyunsaturated fatty acids and depression: When cholesterol does not satisfy. Am J Clin Nutr 1995; 62:1–9.

34. Passwater, RA. Evening primrose oil. In Barilla, J. ed. The Nutrition Superbook. New Canaan, Connecticut: Keats Publishing, Inc., 1996:86–87. Passwater cites personal communication with David Horrobin, M.D.

35. Dossey, L. Space, Time, and Medicine. Boston: Shambala, 1985: 216–17.

Chapter Twelve

1. Simopoulos, AT. Omega-3 fatty acids. In Spiller, GE, ed. Handbook of Lipids in Human Nutrition. Boca Raton, Florida: CRC Press, 1996:56.

2. Cunnane, SC. What is the nutritional and clinical significance of alpha-linolenic acid in humans? In Sinclair, A, Gibson, R. eds. Essential Fatty Acids and Eicosanoids. Champaign, Illinois: American Oil Chemists' Society, 1992:179–81.

3. Gibson, RA. What is the best fatty acid composition for the fats of infant formulas? In Sinclair, A, Gibson, R, eds. Essential Fatty Acids and Eicosanoids. Champaign, Illinois: American Oil Chemists' Society, 1992:210–13.

4. Koletzko, B. Is there a need for a dietary supply of both n-3 and n-6 long chain polyunsaturated fatty acid in the perinatal period? In Sinclair, A, Gibson, R, eds. Essential Fatty Acids and Eicosanoids. Champaign, Illinois: American Oil Chemists' Society, 1992:203–09.

5. Kane, P. Personal communication, 1996.

6. Gindin, J, et al. The effect of plant phosphatidylserine on age-associated memory impairment and mood in the functioning elderly. Geriatric Inst for Ed Res, and Department of Geriatrics, Kaplan Hospital, Rhovot, Israel, 1995.

7. Wurtman, RJ, Zeisel, SH. Brain choline: Its sources and effects on the synthesis and release of acetylcholine. Aging 1982;19:303–13.

8. Galli, C, Simopoulos, AP, eds. Dietary n-3 and n-6 fatty acids: Biological effects and nutritional essentiality, Series A; Life Sciences. New York: Plenum Press, 1989:171.

Chapter Thirteen

1. Blaun, R. Psychology Today, May/June, 1996;35–43.
2. Ibid.

Chapter Fourteen

1. Crawford, M, Marsh, D. Nutrition and Evolution. New Canaan, Connecticut: Keats Publishing, 1995:137.
2. Floud, R, Wachter, K, Gregory, A. Height, Health, and History. Cambridge: Cambridge University Press, 1990.
3. Ward, G, Woods, J, Reyzer, M, Salem, N. Artificial rearing of infant rats on milk formula deficient in n-3 essential fatty acids: A rapid method for the production of experimental n-3 deficiency. Lipids 1996;31(1):71–77.
4. Weisinger, HS, Vingrys, AJ, Sinclair, AJ. Dietary manipulations of long-chain polyunsaturate fatty acids in the retina and brain of guinea pigs. Lipids 1995;30:471–73.
5. Simopoulos, AP. Omega-3 fatty acids. In Spiller, GA, ed. Handbook of Lipids in Human Nutrition. Boca Raton, Florida: CRC Press, Inc., 1996:51–73.
6. Rudin, DO. Omega-3 essential fatty acids in medicine. In Bland, JS. 1984–85 Yearbook in Nutritional Medicine. New Canaan, Connecticut: Keats Publishing, Inc., 1985:41.
7. Crawford, MA. The role of dietary fatty acids in biology: Their place in the evolution of the human brain. Nut Rev 1992;11:3–11.
8. Crawford, MA, Cunnane, SC, Harbige, LS. A new theory of evolution: Quantum theory. In Sinclair, A, Gibson, R. (eds). Essential Fatty Acids and Eicosanoids. Champaign, Illinois: American Oil Chemists' Society, 1992:87–95.
9. Stubbs, CD. The structure and function of docosahexaenoic acid in membranes. In Sinclair, A, Gibson, R, eds. Essential Fatty Acids and Eicosanoids. Champaign, Illinois: American Oil Chemists' Society, 1992:116.
10. Crawford, MA, Cunnane, SC, Harbige, LS. A new theory of evolution: Quantum theory. In Sinclair, A, Gibson, R, eds. Essential Fatty Acids and Eicosanoids. Champaign, Illinois: American Oil Chemists' Society, 1992:87–95.

GLOSSARY

Acetylcholine: A neurotransmitter important in mental function, muscle function, and function of the autonomic nervous system.

ALA (alpha-linolenic acid): A long-chain polyunsaturated fatty acid with 18 carbons, three double bonds, in the omega-3 family (18:3n-3). It cannot be manufactured by the human body and, thus, is termed essential.

Alzheimer's disease: A disorder of the brain characterized by declining mental function.

Antioxidant: A substance that protects against free radicals. Some are termed nutritional antioxidants while others are called enzymatic antioxidants.

AA (arachidonic acid): A long-chain polyunsaturated fatty acid from the omega-6 family. AA contains twenty carbons and four double bonds. It is the brain's principal omega-6 fatty acid. Arachidonic acid is found primarily in animal fats and is often too high in modern diets. This fatty acid can be converted into the powerfully inflammatory PGE2 substances. Alpha-linolenic acid, EPA, and DHA can counter the effects of arachidonic acid. GLA from borage or primrose oil is often used to counter the PGE2 substances as well.

ATP (adenosine triphosphate): The energy currency of the body. ATP is used by all cells of the body to carry out their daily activities. The production of this compound is heavily dependent upon dietary nutrients, including fatty acids.

Axons: An extension of the nerve cell that carries the signal away from the nerve cell body to ultimately connect with another nerve cell or a cell of a different type.

Central nervous system: The brain and spinal cord are considered the central nervous system. Nerves that run outside of the skull and spinal column are known as the peripheral nervous system.

Cholesterol: A sterol found in the diet in animal fats. Cholesterol is a vital component of the body's biochemistry used to form steroid hormones such as estrogen, testosterone, and cortisone. The human body makes about 3,000 mg of cholesterol daily—the rough equivalent of one dozen eggs. Roughly one-fourth of the lipids (fatty substances) in myelin occurs as cholesterol.

Choline: A nutritional substance the brain uses to make the neurotransmitter acetylcholine. Choline is sometimes used as a supplement to enhance mental function.

Coenzyme Q10: Also known as ubiquinone, CoQ10 is a nutrient that serves two primary functions. It is an antioxidant and also functions as a key nutrient in mitochondrial generation of ATP. Thus, CoQ10 is very important in brain energy production.

Cytochrome P450: A system of enzymes the body uses to detoxify foreign or harmful chemicals.

Degenerative disease: The gradual deterioration of a body system that results in the expression of symptoms.

Delta-5-desaturase: The enzyme that converts omega-6 fatty acids such as linoleic acid and GLA into arachidonic acid. High carbohydrate diets may activate this enzyme causing the body to make too much arachidonic acid. This feeds the inflammatory pathways.

Delta-6-desaturase: The enzyme that converts dietary linoleic acid to PGE1. It also converts alpha-linolenic to PGE3. This enzyme is needed to make DHA from ALA. Linoleic acid and linolenic acid compete for delta-6-desaturase so if there is too much of one fatty acid, the products of that fatty acid predominate.

Dendrite: An extension of the nerve cell that receives an impulse and carries it back to the nerve cell body.

Dendritic branches: Like the branches of a tree, they project off the main dendrite. Increased branching allows for greater communication between nerve cells.

Dendritic spines: Tiny structures that project off the dendrite or dendritic branch. They increase the number of synaptic connections that each neuron can make with other neurons. This increases the efficiency with which various regions of the body communicate with one another. There can be literally thousands of dendritic spines, allowing for up to 20,000 synapses with other nerve cells.

DHA (docosahexaenoic acid): A long-chain polyunsaturated fatty derived from dietary alpha-linolenic acid. DHA is also found in foods such as salmon, mackerel, herring, and sardines. It contains twenty-two carbons, six double bonds, and is an omega-3 fatty acid. This is written 22:6n-3. DHA is the most-important omega-3 fatty acid found in the brain and is highly concentrated in the retina.

DNA (deoxyribonucleic acid): The genetic material that exists in the nucleus of all cells. DNA provides the blueprint or model for all body functions. It is very sensitive to damage by free radicals.

Enzymes: Proteins that induce changes in biochemical systems. Practically, they assist in changing one substance into something else. For example, delta-6-desaturase helps to add double bonds into fatty acid molecules making them more unsaturated. It converts alpha-linolenic acid to EPA. Another enzyme then converts EPA into the brain-fat DHA. Enzymes usually require vitamins and minerals as cofactors and catalysts.

EPA (eicosapentaenoic acid): A long-chain polyunsaturated fatty acid derived from dietary alpha-linolenic acid. It contains twenty carbons, five double bonds, and is an omega-3 fatty acid. EPA can be made into PGE3, an anti-inflammatory substance that helps counter the effects of the inflammatory PGE2 substances. EPA is not found in the brain, but can be converted into DHA for use in the brain. EPA is important in the brain's blood supply.

Free radical: A highly reactive molecule, atom, or molecular fragment that has a free or unpaired electron. Free radicals react quickly with protein, fat, and carbohydrate in the body. They are also capable of reacting with almost any cell or tissue causing damage. Free radicals are essential to the function of the human body. Problems occur when free-radical production begins to exceed the body's ability to protect against them. This occurs in many disease processes. Antioxidants protect against free radicals. The highly unsaturated fatty acids in the brain are especially sensitive to free radicals.

Free radical reaction: A reaction in which a free radical reacts with a molecule.

Ginkgo biloba: An herb derived from one of the oldest trees on the planet. This herb is a potent stimulant of cerebral circulation. It is helpful in preventing senile changes in old age.

GLA (gamma-linolenic acid): A long-chain polyunsaturated fatty acid from the omega-6 family. It is used as a supplement to increase production of the body's PGE1 anti-inflammatory system. It is also used when the enzyme delta-6-desaturase is thought to be blocked. GLA should be used with great caution (under supervision of a physician) in cases of seizure or cancer.

Glycemic index: The potential of a sugar or carbohydrate to raise blood sugar levels. High glycemic index foods tend to raise insulin levels higher. High insulin may stimulate the conversion of omega-6 fatty acids into the inflammatory arachidonic acid.

Glutathione: A sulfur-containing nutritional antioxidant. It helps protect the body from free-radical damage. Glutathione is also important in the body's detoxification process. Glutathione stores in the brain become depleted in some brain disorders and in aging.

Glutathione peroxidase: An enzymatic antioxidant that is dependent upon the trace element selenium.

LA (linoleic acid): One of the *essential* fatty acids, meaning the human body cannot make it. LA is written 18:2n-6, meaning is has eighteen carbons, two double bonds, and is of the omega-6 family. It must be obtained from the diet. Modern diets often contain too much linoleic acid relative to other fatty acids.

Leukotriene: A highly inflammatory substance made from arachidonic acid. The body needs this substance, but problems occur when too much is produced.

Lecithin: Also known as phosphatidylcholine. See PC.

Lipid: A general term used to describe fatty molecules derived from the diet. Fatty acids, triglycerides, phospholipids, and waxes are included in this group. Cholesterol is technically not a fat, but a sterol. However, it is still considered a lipid.

Lipid peroxide: A damaged fatty acid (or other lipid) molecule that develops when free radicals or free oxygen react with an unsaturated fatty acid. Lipid peroxides are very damaging to biological systems, especially the cell membrane. Lipid peroxides in the nervous system are very detrimental. Lipid peroxides are also found in rancid oils. Thus, one might think of lipid peroxides in the body as rancid fats.

Mitochondria: Tiny "organelles" within the cell that act as energy factories. This is where the body takes the fuel provided by diet and converts it into the energy that drives every process in the body.

Monounsaturated fat: An unsaturated fatty acid that contains one double bond.

Nerve: A cell that carries information to and from the central nervous system.

Nerve growth factor: A substance that stimulates the growth of neurons.

Neural fat: Fats that are important in the structure and function of the nervous system.

Neurotransmitter: A substance, often a protein or amino acid, which facilitates communication between cells in the nervous system. They affect such things as mood, behavior, thirst, hunger, sleep, muscle contraction, and other actions. In the receptor interaction, the neurotransmitter is like the ship that must fit in the appropriately-shaped dock.

Norepinephrine: A neurotransmitter involved in aggression, alertness, and concentration. It is made from the dietary amino acids tyrosine and phenylalanine.

Omega designation: A term used to describe fatty acid families based on the position of the first double bond. Three categories are generally recognized: omega-3, omega-6, and omega-9. Numeric terms help identify the length of the fatty acid, the number of double bonds, and the position of the first double bond. The fatty acid DHA, for example, is written in numeric terms as 22:6n-3, which means it has twenty-two carbons, six double bonds, and is in the omega-3 family.

Omega-6 to Omega-3 ratio: A comparison of the amount of omega-6 fatty acids to omega-3 fatty acids. Ancient diets were estimated to contain a 1:1 ratio. Modern diets contain as high as a 30:1 ratio.

Oxidation: A biochemical reaction in which an electron is removed from a compound. The opposite of oxidation is called reduction. Whenever something is oxidized something else is reduced. Oxygen is a common molecule that participates in oxidation reactions. Brain fatty acids are highly susceptible to damage by oxidation.

Parkinson's disease: A degenerative disease of the nervous system in which the portion of the brain that secretes dopamine is slowly destroyed. When this occurs, movement is poorly controlled resulting in tremors and weakness.

Peripheral nervous system: That portion of the nervous system outside the skull and spinal cord that supplies, for example, the skin, limbs, and the organs of the abdominal cavity.

PC, phosphatidylcholine. A component of the nerve cell membrane made up of two fatty acids, phosphate, and choline. Also known as lecithin. High in eggs and soy. It is used as a supplement in a number of brain disorders.

PE, phosphatidylethanolamine. A component of the nerve cell membrane made up of two fatty acids, phosphate, and ethanolamine.

PI, phosphatidylinositol. A component of the nerve cell membrane made up of two fatty acids, phosphate, and inositol.

PS, phosphatidylserine. A component of the nerve cell membrane made up of two fatty acids, phosphate, and serine. PS has been used as a supplement in a number of brain disorders.

Platelet: Tiny, microscopic cells that cluster together to form clots. Platelets clump together to plug wounded vessels when the skin is cut, for example. Platelet clumping is influenced by chemical messengers in the blood. Prostacyclin reduces platelet stickiness, thromboxane increases platelet stickiness. When platelets gather and clump within the blood vessels, they can impair blood flow to the brain. Fatty acids strongly influence platelet clumping.

Prostacyclin: A chemical messenger that relaxes blood vessels and prevents platelets from sticking together excessively. Prostacyclin production is encouraged by omega-3 fatty acids, magnesium, and other factors.

Prostaglandins: Hormonelike substances that are derived from fatty acids. Some are strongly inflammatory, while others tend to be anti-inflammatory. Beyond this, they have many other functions in the body. The most commonly described prostaglandins include:

PGE1: made from LA and GLA; is anti-inflammatory
PGE2: made from AA; is a powerful inflammatory substance
PGE3: made from ALA; is mildly anti-inflammatory

Receptors: Sites on the surface of cells where hormones, neurotransmitters, and other substances can attach. Receptors can be likened to a dock into which a ship of a very specific shape must fit. They are of a specific size and shape necessary to react very specifically to another molecule. When a molecule attaches to a receptor the nerve signal can be sent. Receptors are strongly influenced by the fatty-acid structure of the cell membrane.

Saturated fat: Fat molecules that contain no double bonds. The body can easily make these so they are not dietarily essential. Excess saturated fat in the diet can impair the production of neural fatty acids and therefore adversely affect the brain.

Stroke: Is also called "brain attack" in the modern vernacular. It is a rupture or narrowing of blood vessels in the brain leading to damage in the area the vessel normally supplies.

Superoxide dismutase (SOD): An antioxidant enzyme that neutralizes the superoxide free radical. The enzyme requires zinc and copper. In mitochondria, the enzyme requires manganese.

Synapse: The gap between nerve cells. It is the point where the bulb-shaped tip of one neuron abuts the bulb, shaft, or spine of another neuron. A tiny gap exists between them, which allows for the flow of neurotransmitters and other substances. The synaptic membranes of the neuron are highly concentrated with DHA. DHA deficiency adversely affects function of the synapse. The synapse is critical to all nerve cell communication.

Thromboxane: A chemical messenger that causes blood vessels to spasm and platelets to clump. It is formed from the fatty acid arachidonic acid.

Trans fatty acid: An unsaturated fatty acid that has been altered in a way that cause a flip-flop at the position of the double bond. This changes the fatty acid from its normal curved shape to a arrow shape. These harmful fats are more likely to be solid at body temperature, they change cell membrane fluidity, and have been found to enter the brain in animal studies. These undesirable fats should be avoided.

Unsaturated fat: Fats that contain double-bonds between their carbon atoms in one or more locations. Common dietary fats linoleic and linolenic acid contain two and three points of unsaturation, or double bonds. DHA is a highly unsaturated fatty acid containing six double bonds. Those with higher number of double bonds are more susceptible to damage and require greater antioxidant protection.

INDEX

244

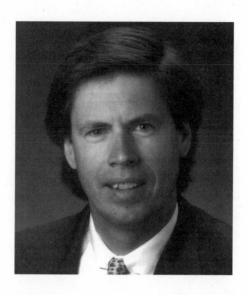

Michael A. Schmidt is a Fellow at the Functional Medicine Research Center (HealthComm, Intl.) in Gig Harbor, Washington, working in the area of clinical nutrition and functional medicine. He is a Visiting Professor of Applied Biochemistry and Clinical Nutrition at Northwestern College, and lectures in Brain Biochemistry and Nutritional Neuroscience. He has written and lectured extensively on the influence of mind, nutrition, and environment on the immune system, and on general health. Dr. Schmidt is the author of several popular books on the subject of integrated medicine, including *Beyond Antibiotics*, a Health Book-of-the-Month Featured Selection.